Department of Health
The Scottish Office Department of Health
Welsh Office
Department of Health and Social Services,
Northern Ireland

Drug Misuse and Dependence – Guidelines on Clinical Management

London: TSO

Published by TSO (The Stationery Office) and available from:

Online
www.tso.co.uk/bookshop

Mail, Telephone, Fax & E-mail
TSO
PO Box 29, Norwich, NR3 1GN
Telephone orders/General enquiries: 0870 600 5522
Fax orders: 0870 600 5533
E-mail: book.orders@tso.co.uk
Textphone 0870 240 3701

TSO Shops
123 Kingsway, London, WC2B 6PQ
020 7242 6393 Fax 020 7242 6394
68-69 Bull Street, Birmingham B4 6AD
0121 236 9696 Fax 0121 236 9699
9-21 Princess Street, Manchester M60 8AS
0161 834 7201 Fax 0161 833 0634
16 Arthur Street, Belfast BT1 4GD
028 9023 8451 Fax 028 9023 5401
18-19 High Street, Cardiff CF10 1PT
029 2039 5548 Fax 029 2038 4347
71 Lothian Road, Edinburgh EH3 9AZ
0870 606 5566 Fax 0870 606 5588

TSO Accredited Agents
(see Yellow Pages)

and through good booksellers

Published with the permission of the
Department of Health on behalf of
the Controller of her Majesty's Stationery Office.

First published 1999
Fourth impression 2006

ISBN O 11 322277 7

Printed in the United Kingdom for The Stationery Office

184601 C15 1/06

CONTENTS

Chapter 2
Treatment

Chapter 3
Assessment

Chapter 4
The responsibilities and principles of prescribing for drug dependence

Chapter 5
The management of dependence and withdrawal

Chapter 6
Dose reduction regimens

Chapter 7
Preventing relapse

Annex 1
Shared working with other professionals

Annex 2
Training for clinicians working with drug misusers

Annex 3
Health and safety/managing challenging behaviour

Annex 4
Models of change

Annex 5
Pregnancy and neonatal care

Annex 6
Young people and drugs

Annex 7
HIV, Hepatitis B and C

Annex 8
Alcohol and drug misuse

Annex 9
The criminal justice system

Annex 10
Accident and emergency

Annex 11
Mental health

Annex 12
Harm minimisation for injecting drug misusers

Annex 13
How to write a prescription for a controlled drug

Annex 14
Drug interactions – methadone drug interactions

Annex 15
Conversion table

Annex 16
Drugs and driving

Annex 17
Travelling abroad

Annex 18
Monitoring progress and outcomes of treatment

Annex 19
References and contact numbers

Membership of the Clinical Guidelines on Drug Misuse and Dependence Working Group

Chairman

Professor John Strang

Director of the National Addiction Centre.
The Chief Medical Officer's Clinical Adviser on Drug Misuse. A member of the Advisory Council on the Misuse of Drugs.

Members

1.   Psychiatrists

Dr Eilish Gilvarry
Consultant Psychiatrist and former GP. Clinical Director of Northern Alcohol and Drug Service, Newcastle upon Tyne. Co-author HAS report on *Alcohol and Drug Services for Young People*. Member of Joint RCPsych/RCGP Committee on Shared Care.

Dr Philip Fleming
Consultant Psychiatrist, Drug and Alcohol Service, Portsmouth Health Care Trust. Member of SCODA Executive Committee. Recent research on amphetamine prescribing and GP training.

Dr Duncan Raistrick
Consultant Psychiatrist, Leeds Addiction Centre. CMO's Clinical Adviser on Alcohol Misuse. Research on methadone and GP training.

Dr Diana Patterson
Consultant Psychiatrist in Belfast. A member of the Advisory Council on the Misuse of Drugs. Chair of the Northern Ireland Committee on Drug Misuse.

Dr Mary Rowlands
Former Senior Medical Officer, HM Prison, Bristol. Active in developing drug treatment in HM Prison Service. Member of 1991 Clinical Guidelines Group.

Dr David Curson
Consultant Psychiatrist at the Roehampton Priory Hospital. Member of the BUPA consensus panel in psychiatry.

2.   General practitioners

Dr Clare Gerada

GP in South London. GP consultant of a primary care liaison drug service. Published numerous articles and book chapters on primary care aspects of addictions. Honorary Senior Lecturer, Department of Psychiatry, King's College Hospital. Joined the Department of Health, March 1998, as a Senior Policy Adviser.

Dr Christine Ford

GP in north-west London, GP facilitator for substance misuse in Brent and Harrow HA (and Clinical Director of Brent Specialist Drug and Alcohol Services, since April 1998). Chair of organising committee of annual conference on managing drug users in general practice. GP drugs specialist with experience of prescribing injectable methadone.

Dr William Clee

GP drugs specialist in Cardiff. Experience of Welsh amphetamine problem. A member of the Advisory Council on the Misuse of Drugs. Newly appointed Chairman of Welsh Advisory Committee on Drug and Alcohol Misuse.

Dr Judy Bury

Primary care facilitator for HIV and drugs in Edinburgh, previously a GP. Developed *Managing Drug Users in General Practice*, a handbook widely used in Scotland. Co-worker of Dr Judy Greenwood's at pioneering Lothian service for shared care of drug users.

3.   Public health

Dr Laurence Gruer

Consultant in public health medicine with Greater Glasgow Health Board. Responsible for planning and implementing a wide range of drug misuse services, including a large city-wide methadone programme involving GPs, community pharmacists and community drugs services. A member of the Advisory Council on the Misuse of Drugs and the Scottish Advisory Committee on Drug Misuse.

Dr Sally Hargreaves

Director of Public Health, Kensington and Chelsea and Westminster Health Authority. Interested in shared care and private practice issues in her HA. Direct involvement in drug misuse purchasing.

4.   Nursing

Professor Jean Faugier

Nursing specialist in drug misuse treatment. Currently at NW regional office of the NHS Executive. Ex Chairman of ANSA (Association of Nurses in Substance Abuse). Visiting Professor of Nursing at Department of Nursing, Liverpool.

5.   Pharmacists

Dr Janie Sheridan
Senior Research Pharmacist, currently at the National Addiction Centre. Has undertaken important research on prescribing pattern of methadone in NHS and private practice, and on the role of the pharmacist in service provision to drug misusers.

6.   Non-statutory agencies

Mr Roger Howard
Chief Executive of Standing Conference on Drug Abuse (SCODA). A member of the Advisory Council on the Misuse of Drugs.

7.   Accident and emergency medicine

Professor John Henry
Professor of Accident and Emergency at St Mary's Hospital, Paddington. Clinical pharmacologist. An authority on Ecstasy (MDMA).

8.   General Medical Council representative

Professor Andrew Sims
Division of Psychiatry and Behavioural Sciences, St James' University Hospital, Leeds.

Observers

Alan Macfarlane
Home Office Drugs Inspectorate

Dr John Loudon
Scottish Home and Health Department

Dr Sarah Watkins
Welsh Office

Dr Glenda Mock
Department of Health and Social Services, Northern Ireland

Dr Somasundan
HM Prison Service Health Care Directorate

Stephen Rimmer/John Cairncross
Central Drugs Coordination Unit /UK Anti-Drugs Coordination Unit

Secretariat

Dr Michael Farrell – Department of Health
Dr Anthony Thorley – Department of Health
Rosemary Jenkins – Department of Health
Fred Pink – Department of Health

FOREWORD

Previous Guidelines

Drug Misuse and Dependence: Guidelines on Clinical Management was last revised in 1991. Substantial changes in the extent and patterns of misuse and developments in treatment have required a revision of the Guidelines and a new approach to their structure and content.

A Working Group was set up in January 1997 by the Department of Health to revise the 1991 Guidelines. Professor John Strang was invited by the Chief Medical Officer to chair the Group. The broad multidisciplinary membership of the Group reflects the increasing number of professionals involved in the clinical management of drug misuse and dependence, and the need for a wider community perspective on the treatment of drug misusers.

Terms of reference

The terms of reference of the group were to revise the document *Drug Misuse and Dependence: Guidelines on Clinical Management* in the light of developments since 1991, particularly:

    i)   the policy implications of *Tackling Drugs Together*, and the equivalent strategies in Scotland, Wales and Northern Ireland;

    ii)   the emergence of new patterns of drug misuse;

    iii)   new developments in treatment, rehabilitation and prevention;

These Guidelines make a number of recommendations (e.g. those on supervised consumption), which for practical reasons, may need to be phased in over a time period in some cases.

These Guidelines will be subject to future review as appropriate.

Who are the Guidelines for?

These Guidelines are written for all doctors. They are intended for those doctors who are 'generalists' in the sense that they do not have any particular expertise in drug misuse (e.g. general practitioners, physicians, surgeons and obstetricians); and for those practitioners who have varying degrees of training and expertise treating drug misusers, including specialists in drug misuse and some general practitioners. The distribution of the Guidelines will include, amongst others, all GPs, Accident and Emergency consultants, NHS trusts, health authorities and specialist drug treatment centres. They will also be available on the Department of Health's web site at **www.doh.gov.uk/drugdep.htm**.

What the Guidelines *do not* cover

These Guidelines are not a comprehensive textbook or manual for the treatment of drug misuse. Doctors and other professionals should access more detailed information and specialist advice about interventions described in the Guidelines.[1]

For the purpose of these Guidelines, treatment is divided into assessment, management of withdrawal and dependence, and preventing relapse.

The nature of the Guidelines

These Guidelines have been developed within the framework for guidelines development, supported by the Department of Health in conjunction with professional bodies. This framework is set out in the good practice booklet *Clinical Guidelines: Using Clinical Guidelines to improve patient care within the NHS.*

Unlike other clinical guidelines, these have been funded and published by the Department of Health itself, rather than a professional body. This is because clinical interventions for drug misuse and dependence are subject to a number of regulations for the prescribing of controlled drugs.

Evidence-based Guidelines

The Guidelines are based on a number of sources of evidence for effectiveness. They are primarily based on evidence obtained from expert committee reports and the clinical experience of respected authorities. Written evidence was sought and received from a wide range of medical and non-medical bodies, and individual professionals working in this field. These included the Royal College of General Practitioners, the Royal College of Psychiatrists and the Royal Pharmaceutical Society of Great Britain.

Given the broad range of clinical topics covered and the variable level of the evidence available, this Committee has, by a process of consensus, come to a view of the best available evidence from whatever source. It has relied substantially on the major undertaking of the Task Force to review services for drug misusers.[2] The Committee has attempted to incorporate all significant published evidence that has occurred since then. In the context of the process of systematic reviewing there is currently, with some exceptions, a limited amount of rigorous reviews in this area. We would recommend that systematic reviews be further developed along the lines of the Cochrane Collaboration, and, when they are available, that they be incorporated in a future review of these Clinical Guidelines.

---

[1] Ghodse H. *Drugs and addictive behaviour: a guide to treatment.* Oxford: Blackwell Science, 1995.
[2] Department of Health. *Task Force to review services for drug misusers: report of an Independent Review of Drug Treatment Services in England.* London: Department of Health, 1996. (Chairman: The Reverend Dr John Polkinghorne)

The legal position of the Guidelines

The Guidelines have no defined legal position, except where there are legal obligations in relation to the prescribing of controlled drugs. Doctors need to ensure that they act within Home Office licensing regulations.

However, any doctor not fulfilling the standards and quality of care in the appropriate treatment of drug misusers that are set out in these Clinical Guidelines, will have this taken into account if, for any reason, consideration of their performance in this clinical area is undertaken. A number of bodies can undertake such a consideration of performance.

Since 1997, the General Medical Council has had additional powers, under the Medical (Professional Performance) Act 1995, to take action against any doctor whose professional performance is seriously deficient and possibly putting patients at risk. In that these Guidelines do represent a consensus view of good clinical practice, it is expected that they will be a significant reference point in assisting the General Medical Council in its power to examine reports of alleged poor performance by medical practitioners, in the treatment of drug misuse.

Additionally, the NHS White Papers *The New NHS, Modern, Dependable*[3] in England, *Designed to Care* in Scotland[4], *Putting Patients First* in Wales[5], *Fit for the Future* in Northern Ireland[6], set out the role of a number of measures to achieve quality, nationally and locally. These include a new system of Clinical Governance in NHS Trusts and Primary Care Groups (Local Health Care Co-operatives in Scotland) to ensure that clinical standards are met and that there are processes to ensure continuous quality improvement, backed by a new statutory duty for quality by NHS Trusts. The Commission for Health Improvement will support and oversee the quality of clinical services locally (in England and Wales), and will tackle shortcomings. It will be able to intervene by invitation, or on the Secretary of State's direction, where a problem has not been satisfactorily dealt with.

---

[3] Department of Health. *The new NHS: modern, dependable*. London: The Stationery Office, 1997. (Cm3807)
[4] Scottish Office Department of Health. *Designed to care: renewing the National Health Service in Scotland*. London: The Stationery Office, 1997. (Cm. 3811)
[5] Welsh Office. *NHS Wales: putting patients first*. London: The Stationery Office, 1998. (Cm 3841)
[6] Department of Health and Social Services, Northern Ireland Office. *Fit for the future: a consultation document on the Government's proposals for the future of the health and personal social services in Northern Ireland*. Belfast, Department of Health and Social Services, 1998.

CHAPTER 1
INTRODUCTION

Key chapter recommendations

> **Drug misusers have the same entitlement as other patients to the services provided by the National Health Service. It is the responsibility of all doctors to provide care for both general health needs *and* drug-related problems, whether or not the patient is ready to withdraw from drugs. This should include the provision of evidence-based interventions, such as hepatitis B vaccinations, and providing harm minimisation advice. Every doctor must provide medical care to a standard which could reasonably be expected of that practitioner in his or her position. No practitioner should be put under duress by colleagues or patients to provide treatment beyond that standard unless he or she wishes to.**

1. The growth of drug misuse

Prevalence

The question of how many people are using illicit drugs is deceptively easy to ask but notoriously difficult to answer. The most recent published data from the Regional Drug Misuse Databases[1] show that the total number of drug misusers presenting to treatment in the six months ending March 1998, was around 30,000 in Great Britain. Over half of those users presenting were in their twenties (54 per cent), and around one in seven (15 per cent) were aged under 20. The ratio of males to females was 3:1. Over half (55 per cent) reported heroin as their main drug of misuse. Methadone was the next most frequently reported main drug of misuse with 13 per cent of users, followed by cannabis and amphetamines, both with 9 per cent. Drug misuse is a substantial and growing problem, with a significant and profound impact on the health and social functioning of many individuals. Self-reported drug use amongst those aged 16–59 years in England and Wales in 1996, showed that approximately one in ten had used illegal drugs in the last year, and that one in twenty (6 per cent) had in the last month.[2]

People who are involved in drugs may have multiple social and medical problems. Doctors everywhere must expect to see drug misusers presenting for care and will need to be vigilant in looking for signs of drug misuse in their patients.

Historically, drug misuse has been thought of as an urban problem but this is no longer the case. As there is no easily discernible pattern of drug misuse nationally, so there is a wide range of drug misusers.

---

[1] Department of Health. *Drug misuse statistics for six months ending March 1998*, London: Department of Health, 1999. (Statistical bulletin, 1999/7)

[2] Ramsey M., Spiller J., *Drug misuse declared in 1996: latest results from the British Crime Survey*. London: Home Office, 1997. (Home Office Research Study no. 172)

Young people are increasingly using a wide range of drugs and alcohol at a younger age and the age of initiation into drug use appears to have lowered.[3] There is growing use amongst girls, and polydrug use has become more common as a pattern of misuse. The unclear boundary between so-called 'recreational' drug taking, and drug misuse requiring treatment, highlights the complexity and challenge of the task facing clinicians and services. The typical drug misuser does not exist. Each is an individual with his or her own set of problems.

2. Morbidity and mortality

Misusers of some types of drugs are at an increased risk of death compared with their non-drug misusing counterparts. A long-term follow-up of heroin addicts showed they had a mortality risk nearly twelve times greater than the general population.[4] Another study of injecting drug misusers showed that they were twenty-two times more likely to die than their non-injecting peers.[5] Recent research in the UK has shown that from 1985–1995 there was a marked increase in drug-related deaths amongst young people, aged 15–19 years.[6] Mortality from self-poisoning with opiates has increased over ninefold in the past two decades.[7] The high morbidity and mortality rates make it particularly important that drug misusers are in contact with treatment services.

3. Rights and responsibilities

In addition, a doctor must guard against personal prejudice colouring clinical attitude and practice. The General Medical Council has stated:

> *"It is . . . unethical for a doctor to withhold treatment from any patient on the basis of a moral judgement that the patient's activities or lifestyle might have contributed to the condition for which treatment was being sought. Unethical behaviour of this kind may raise the question of serious professional misconduct."*

All individuals are entitled to the same standard and range of treatments, as set out in these Guidelines.

Health Authorities, Primary Care Groups and future Primary Care Trusts in England and Wales, Health Boards in Northern Ireland and Scotland, and Local Health Care Cooperatives in Scotland, all have a duty to provide treatment for drug misusers.

All GPs treating individuals for drug misuse have a right to support from their Health Authority or relevant primary care organisation.

---

[3] Parker H., Measham F., Aldridge J., *Drugs Futures: changing patterns of drug use amongst English youth*. London: Institute for the Study of Drug Dependence, 1995. (ISDD research monograph 7)

[4] Oppenheimer E., Tobutt C., Taylor C., Andrew T., 'Death and survival in a cohort of heroin addicts from London clinics: a 22-year, follow-up study', *Addiction* 1994; **89**: 1299–1308.

[5] Frischer M., Goldberg D., Rahman M., Bemey L., 'Mortality and survival amongst a cohort of drug injectors in Glasgow 1982–1994', *Addiction* 1997; **92**: 419-427.

[6] Roberts I., Barker M., Li L. 'Analysis of trends in deaths from accidental drug poisoning in teenagers 1985–1995', *British Medical Journal* 1997; **315**: 289.

[7] Neeleman I., Farrell M., 'Fatal methadone and heroin overdoses: time trends in England and Wales.' *Journal of Epidemiol Community Health* 1997; **51**: 435–437.

4. The changing organisation of primary care

At the time of publication of these Guidelines, the organisation of primary care is undergoing considerable change. The basic tenet of an independent practitioner, working alone or in partnerships, from purpose-built or modified premises, is still in operation. However, the introduction of Primary Care Groups and their equivalents, together with joint working within and outside the profession, and the formation of Primary Care Trusts, will undoubtedly affect the delivery and organisation of primary (and secondary) care. New initiatives such as the introduction of salaried options for GPs in England (Primary Care Act pilots), Section 36 funding (Section 37 in Scotland), Local Development Schemes, nurse prescribing, Health Action Zones (there are none in Scotland), and GP commissioning pilots mean that new ways are available to deliver services to patients.

5. The new policy agenda

Two publications provide a framework for current drug treatment policy in England. Separate strategies exist in Scotland and Wales, which adhere to the same basic principles.

a) The Effectiveness Review (1996)[8]

The Task Force to Review Services for Drug Misusers recommended that all drug misusers need to have access to primary care through normal registration with a GP and that GPs are well placed to identify and offer advice to drug misusers who may not be in touch with specialist agencies.

The Review identified a dual role for GPs in the treatment of drug misuse: the provision of general medical services and the provision of care and treatment for drug misuse, including the identification of drug misuse; where appropriate, referral to specialist drug services; promoting harm minimisation; and undertaking shared care with a service specialising in the treatment of drug misuse. The Review recommended that the provision of shared care, with appropriate support for GPs, should be available as widely as possible.

b) Tackling Drugs to Build a Better Britain (1998)[9]

The new Drugs Strategy, 'Tackling Drugs to Build a Better Britain', identifies treatment as one of its four key elements, and recognises that there is growing evidence that treatment works.

The strategy aims to:

> *"enable people with drug problems to overcome them and to live healthy and crime-free lives."*

---

[8] Department of Health. *Task Force to review services for drug misusers: report of an Independent Review of Drug Treatment Services in England.* London: Department of Health, 1996. (Chairman: The Reverend Dr John Polkinghorne)
[9] *Tackling drugs to build a better Britain: the Government's ten-year strategy for tackling drug misuse.* London: The Stationery Office, 1998. (Cm 3945)

This means ensuring that:

> " . . . *all problem drug misusers – irrespective of age, gender, race and drug of choice – have proper access to support from appropriate services – including primary care . . .*"

Activity which springs from the strategy:

> " . . . *will ensure that prescription of substitute medications in particular and the dispensing of clinical services in general are in line with forthcoming Department of Health Clinical Guidelines.*"

6. The generalist, specialised generalist and specialist

These Guidelines recognise that the management and treatment of drug misusers present medical practitioners with particular challenges. The range and complexity of treatment and rehabilitation produces the need for a continuum of medical practice, skills and experience, ranging from the contribution that can be made by all doctors to that made by specialised practitioners. The Guidelines also acknowledge the importance placed on treating drug misuse in a primary care setting, which is often seen as less stigmatising than specialised agencies. Involving GPs in the care of drug misuse and expansion of shared care is not seen as an alternative to the current role of the specialist services. Some drug misusers will continue to need specialist support which it would be unreasonable to expect a GP to provide in general practice. GPs should, however, be sufficiently skilled to identify a problem drug misuser, who is consulting them for other, perhaps related problems. This is likely to require a programme of training for GPs.

For the purpose of these Guidelines, and in order to recognise the expansion of specialisation within a generalist setting, three levels of expertise are described: the generalist, the specialised generalist and the specialist. The terms 'specialist' and 'specialised generalist' are intended to be helpful and descriptive, they should not be considered as representing legal entities. It should be noted that these levels are not meant to be prescriptive, although many doctors will recognise their practice within them. They represent a continuum by which the development of shared care arrangements, training, provision of resources and Home Office licensing arrangements can be targeted. Whatever service a doctor is offering within this continuum, he/she must ensure they are trained to a competence commensurate with that activity. The three levels of care can apply to all doctors whether in the NHS or private practice, be they general practitioners, hospital specialists or doctors whose main expertise is in the area of drug misuse.

Level 1: the generalist

Generalists are medical practitioners who may be involved in the treatment of drug misuse, although this is not their main area of work. They should be able to demonstrate relevant competence to underpin their practice and care for a number of drug misusers, usually on a shared care basis. Services to be provided would be expected to include the assessment of drug misusers and, where appropriate, the prescribing of substitute medication.

All these services would normally be carried out with the provision of support from a shared care scheme or following the advice from a more suitably experienced medical practitioner (specialist or specialised generalist). Practitioners would be encouraged to enter into a locally agreed treatment scheme or guideline to ensure consistent standards and integrated care.

Such doctors would undergo regular training and have knowledge of prescribing issues and options, approaches to the development and understanding of dependence, policy issues and the management of drug treatment.

Level 2: the specialised generalist

A specialised generalist is a practitioner whose work is essentially generic or, if a specialist, is not primarily concerned with drug misuse treatment, but who has a specicial interest in treating drug misusers. Such practitioners would have expertise and competence to provide assessment of most cases with complex needs.

Examples of a specialised generalist would be a general practitioner or a prison medical officer who deals with large numbers of drug misusers in their practice and who, with other professionals and agencies, provides many of the services that are necessary. Their drug misuse practice would possibly involve prescription of specialised drug regimens. Additionally, they can potentially act as an expert resource in shared care arrangements for general practitioners and professional staff operating at Level 1.

Such doctors would be required to undergo appropriate training to enable them to maintain this level of competence.

Level 3: the specialist

A specialist is a practitioner who provides expertise, training and competence in drug misuse treatment as their main clinical activity. Such a practitioner works in a specialist multidisciplinary team, can carry out assessment of any case with complex needs and provide a full range of treatments and access to rehabilitation options.

Most specialists would normally (but not always) be a consultant psychiatrist who holds a Certificate of Completion of Specialist Training (CCST) in psychiatry, and is therefore able to provide expertise, training and competence in drug misuse treatment as their main clinical activity. This data would be held on the specialist register of the General Medical Council. Such doctors would be required to maintain their level of specialist competence by attending appropriate training events.

Their practice would probably involve prescription of injectable and other specialised forms of prescribing, which will require appropriate Home Office licences. They can act as an expert resource in shared care arrangements for other practitioners and professional staff.

Specialists in addiction would hold a higher qualification with a CCST in psychiatry, and would be required to maintain their level of specialist competence by attending appropriate training events.

7. Evidence-based approach to care

In a substantial proportion of patients, drug misuse tends to improve with time and age,[10] particularly when specific treatment and rehabilitation techniques are used. There is also increasing evidence that treatment (medical and social) is effective in maintaining the health of the individual and promoting the process of recovery. Studies of self-recovery by drug users have shown that access to formal welfare supports, together with encouragement from friends, partners, children, parents and other significant individuals, is commonly involved in the pathway out of addiction.[11] Treatment studies do not support the view that a drug user has to reach 'rock-bottom' before being motivated to change. Harm minimisation refers to the reduction of various forms of harm related to drug misuse, including health, social, legal and financial problems, until the drug user is ready and able to come off drugs. A harm minimisation approach improves the public health and social environment by:

---

[10] Thorley A., 'Longitudinal studies of drug dependence', in Edwards, Busch, eds., *Drug problems in Britain: a review of 10 years*. London: Academic Press, 1981; 117–169.

[11] *Treatment works*. Rockville Department of Health and Human Services, 1996.

a) Reducing the risk of infectious diseases and other medical and social harm

There is good evidence that harm minimisation approaches have had considerable success in reducing the rate of Human Immunodeficiency Virus (HIV) among injectors in the drug misusing population.[12]

b) Reducing drug-related deaths

Drug-related deaths can be reduced by:

    i)   engaging and retaining dependent drug misusers in treatment;

    ii)   improving individuals' knowledge of both the risks of overdose, and methods of avoiding overdose.

It is likely that a reduction in diversion of prescribed medicine onto the illegal market would also avoid some drug-related deaths.

c) Reducing criminal activity

Many drug misusers support their drug taking with significant criminal activity, which is both costly and damaging to the individual and wider society. Evidence shows that conventional drug misuse treatment in the UK significantly reduces criminal activity.[13]

---

[12] Stimson G., 'AIDS and injecting drug use in the United Kingdom, 1987-1993: the policy response and the prevention of the epidemic.' *Social Science and Medicine 1995*; **41**: 699–716.
[13] Gossop M., Marsden J., Stewart D., *NTORS at one year: changes in substance use, health and criminal behaviours one year after intake*. London: Department of Health, 1998.

CHAPTER 2
TREATMENT

Key chapter recommendations

Medical practitioners should not prescribe in isolation but should seek to liaise with other professionals who will be able to help with factors contributing to an individual's drug misuse. A multidisciplinary approach to treatment is therefore essential.

Where there are no local specialist services with which a shared care agreement can be developed, it is the responsibility of the health authority to ensure that appropriate services are in place. This might mean, for example, developing a shared care arrangement with a service in the independent or private sector or providing support for primary care practices to develop as secondary providers i.e. specialised generalists. The guiding principle is that support for GPs should include expert prescribing advice and guidance on medico-legal matters, and be grounded in knowledge and experience of treating more complex cases (e.g. polydrug dependence, pregnant drug misusers and those with a mental illness).

1. Aims of treatment

■ Assist the patient to remain healthy, until, with appropriate care and support, he or she can achieve a drug-free life.

■ Reduce the use of illicit or non-prescribed drugs by the individual.

■ Deal with problems related to drug misuse.

■ Reduce the dangers associated with drug misuse, particularly the risk of HIV, hepatitis B and C, and other blood-borne infections from injecting and sharing injecting paraphernalia.

■ Reduce the duration of episodes of drug misuse.

■ Reduce the chance of future relapse to drug misuse.

■ Reduce the need for criminal activity to finance drug misuse.

■ Reduce the risk of prescribed drugs being diverted onto the illegal drug market.

■ Stabilise the patient where appropriate on a substitute medication to alleviate withdrawal symptoms.

■ Improve overall personal, social and family functioning.

2. The treatment setting: shared care and multidisciplinary working

Some patients present with complex needs: risk of HIV and other blood-borne viruses, comorbid physical or psychiatric illness, a forensic history, problems with personal relationships, employment and housing. This demands effective collaboration between medical practitioners (e.g. GPs, obstetricians and gynaecologists, general psychiatrists and prison medical officers), specialist drug misuse treatment services, social services voluntary sector and the criminal justice system.

Shared care is a model that can be applied to any close cooperative work between agencies or services, which directly improves the treatment of the individual drug misuser. It most often involves arrangements between specialist and general practitioner services. However, a multidisciplinary approach necessitates shared working across, and between, a number of different agencies and professionals within the drugs field and beyond.

The Department of Health defines shared care as "The joint participation of specialists and GPs (and other agencies as appropriate) in the planned delivery of care for patients with a drug misuse problem, informed by an enhanced information exchange beyond routine discharge and referral letters. It may involve the day-to-day management by the GP of the patient's medical needs in relation to his or her drug misuse. Such arrangements would make explicit which clinician was responsible for different aspects of the patient's treatment and care. These may include prescribing substitute drugs in appropriate circumstances." [1]

A number of specific factors and features, relevant to the treatment of drug misusers, account for the development of shared care. They include:

■ Shared care is a rational model to improve service delivery: it aims to deliver a flexible service, utilising differing skills in the most effective manner.[2]

■ The general shift towards a better balance of primary and secondary health care provision with the emphasis being placed on a primary-care-led NHS.

■ An increasing preference by drug misusers to receive care in a primary care setting in the community wherever possible.

---

[1] *Reviewed shared care arrangements for drug misusers.* London: Department of Health, 1995 (Executive letter; EL(95) 114).
[2] Gask L., Sibbald B., Creed F., 'Evaluating models of working at the interface between mental health services and primary care'. *British Journal of Psychiatry* 1997; 170: 6–11.

■   Expansion of the primary health care team to include a wide range of specialist mental health staff, including community psychiatric nurses, clinical psychologists, and specialist drug and alcohol workers.

■   The increasing number of young drug misusers whose natural first point of contact is their family doctor.

Shared care is not limited solely to prescribing issues. It should be seen as part of a range of treatment options that can be offered[3], which include:

■   interventions to support drug misusers who wish to give up without a need for prescribing;

■   specific treatment interventions (e.g. counselling, non-pharmacological therapies);

■   interventions carried out between general practice and voluntary drug agencies.

a) The role of the general practitioner in shared care[4]

Shared care should not be perceived as a panacea for all the challenges faced by services in providing good clinical practice for the treatment of drug misuse. Indeed, it is not always appropriate for many patients to be managed within a shared care model. Some should be managed principally by specialist services, whether voluntary agencies or a specialist medical drug misuse treatment clinic, and some mainly by the general practitioner, and a conventional level of liaison and communication should take place. However, all patients should be strongly encouraged to receive their general medical care from a general practitioner.

It follows that good practice, utilising shared care, places a great emphasis on developing close links between the primary health care team and specific specialist staff, in order to:

■   *Enhance* general practitioner skills in the detection and management of patients with drug misuse problems;

■   *Reduce* referrals to the specialist services for patients with less complex medical needs and problems and hence enable the patient to be treated in primary care for as long as possible;

■   *Encourage* selective referrals to specialist services for patients with more complex needs and problems.

[3] Gerada C., Farrell M., 'Shared care', in: Robertson R., ed., *Management of drug users in the community: a practical handbook*. Arnold, 1998; 328–352.

[4] Elander J., Porter S., Hodson S., 'What role for general practitioners in the care of opiate users?' *Addiction Research* 1994; **1**: 309–322.

b) The role of specialist services in shared care

Shared care can only work well when there is adequate provision of both generalist and specialist services, both in the statutory and voluntary sector.

The expertise of specialist secondary services provided by psychiatric, medical and voluntary agencies would be expected when dealing with the following situations:

- Patients with serious risk to physical or mental health or complex needs e.g. schizophrenia, liver disease, frequent relapses, polydrug use, concurrent alcohol misuse, complications of drug misuse or a chaotic lifestyle.

- Patients with a serious forensic history.

- Patients not responding to oral substitute prescribing, who may require less frequently used interventions such as injectable opioids, should in most circumstances be managed by a specialist service.

- Patients requiring a large element of psychosocial therapy or support for housing, employment and training.

- Patients requiring specialised in-patient or day care.

- Patients requiring a specialist residential rehabilitation programme.

c) Shared care guidelines

There is no single ideal model of shared care. Different areas will have different needs depending on geographical variables, available expertise in primary and secondary care, and numbers of drug misusers and the provision of treatment facilities.[5] In some cases shared care may take the form of a dedicated team from a specific agency, e.g. a community drug team. The appointment of a liaison or link worker can facilitate shared care to one or more GP practices. The key to success lies in the level of specialist support available to the GP and Primary Health Care Team, ease of access to this support, and the willingness and flexibility of all parties involved in shared care to work together. In all situations the multiple needs of the patient should not be jeopardised by poor co-ordination and communication.

The development of local shared care guidelines is essential: they should take account of national policy, but be locally determined, so as to incorporate the range of options for local service. The drawing up of guidelines should involve all provider participants, including general practitioners (generalists and specialised generalists), specialists, pharmacists and voluntary agencies.

---

[5] Gerada C., Tighe, J., 'A review of shared care protocols for the treatment of problem drug use in England, Scotland and Wales.' *The British Journal of General Practice* 1999; **439**: 125–6.

Guidelines might specifically incorporate:

- standardised assessment, treatment and referral protocols;

- roles and responsibilities of professionals specifically participating in shared care;

- mechanisms for support (e.g. key worker, liaison worker, or, where it has been developed, the shared care team);

- identification of skills, knowledge and training needs, and, importantly, a strategy for how these needs will be implemented;

- agreed monitoring and evaluation arrangements;

- measures to keep abreast of new developments in treatment and rehabilitation, and arrangements to provide a strategic overview on the development of local drug misuse services and patterns of drug misuse (e.g. links to the Drug Action Team).

Drug misusers should have good access to whatever services are available. It is therefore important for every doctor to be aware of local services. Local information may be obtained from the local Drug Action Team, local drug services and from a directory of services such as that held by the Standing Conference On Drug Abuse.[6]

d) Monitoring group

Shared care arrangements are present in some form in all Health Authorities in England and Wales and Health Boards in Scotland and Northern Ireland. However, Primary Care Groups (Local Health Care Co-operatives in Scotland) introducing a more formalised shared care arrangement, including local protocols, as outlined in these guidelines, will need to review existing local service configuration, contracts and researching arrangements for primary and secondary care services.

Progress toward the ideal pattern and delivery of shared care in any area will inevitably be incremental and will rely on developing good communication, understanding and trust between all the services involved. The organisation of effective training for participating personnel and the monitoring of competence will play an important role in achieving success. The development and management of shared care practice is a crucial part of service development for drug misuse and related public health issues at local level over the next few years.

---

[6] See Annex 19 for SCODA's contact number.

It is therefore recommended that a local level shared care monitoring group be set up. This should relate to the Drug Action Team, and should comprise the Director of Public Health (or deputy), representatives from specialist treatment agencies, general practice, the Local Medical Committee (GP Sub Committee of the Area Medical Committee in Scotland) and other members as required. The monitoring group should agree to approve local agreements and protocols, review training needs, clarify performance indicators and monitor the delivery and effectiveness of shared care service provision in the area.

e) Examples of good practice in shared care of drug misusers

Professional	Role
GP	Treatment of acute episode of illness
	Immunisation
	HIV testing
	Cervical screening
	Family planning advice
	Identification of drug problem*
	Assessment of drug misuse*
	Treatment of drug problems*
	Referral to secondary drug service*
Pharmacist	Daily dispensing of methadone
	Point of contact for general health information
Practice Nurse	Abscess dressing, wound care
Social Worker	Welfare rights, legal advice
Drug Agency	Provision of injecting paraphernalia
	Safer sex advice
	Referral for rehabilitation

*GPs are very likely to require additional training to develop these skills

3. Problems and challenges in multidisciplinary and shared care working

Multidisciplinary and shared care working raise a number of key issues and common dilemmas. In order to optimise clinical and service effectiveness these need to be addressed, and include:

Confidentiality

The place of confidentiality in the context of patient rights, and for the *whole team*, set against differing individual professional requirements. It is important to explore the relationship in a multidisciplinary team between accountability, shared responsibility and individual professional responsibility.

Comprehensive provision

Treatment is not to be seen as simply prescribing a substitute for the drug of dependence, though this is often part of the process. Where a prescription is offered it should form part of a *comprehensive package* to tackle a patient's need, with other services being provided as appropriate.

Clinical practice

The importance for staff in rehabilitation services to acknowledge the need for patients to continue having essential medical and psychiatric medication during treatment and rehabilitation.

Supervision

The need for adequate clinical supervision of team members, and for there to be a framework of supervision which relates, where appropriate, to the overall clinical responsibility of the medical officer. Properly arranged structures for individual staff development, personal support and training must be in place.

Organisational context

Awareness of how the multidisciplinary team fits into a shared care setting.

Role definition

The role of doctors working in voluntary agencies.

A clear policy as to which members of staff have authority to pass on formal clinical advice about substitute prescribing dose levels and regimens to other professionals and agencies.

To clarify these and related issues, it is strongly advised that local guidelines and team policies, which address issues of multidisciplinary working, be devised, understood and implemented by all members of the multidisciplinary team.

CHAPTER 3
ASSESSMENT

Key chapter recommendations

Good assessment is essential to the continuing care of the patient. Not only can it enable the patient to become engaged in treatment but it can begin a process of change even before a full assessment is complete. Assessment skills are vital for all members of the multidisciplinary team, including drugs workers, psychologists, nurses and doctors.

Only in exceptional circumstances should the decision to offer substitute medication without specialised generalist or specialist advice be made. Such examples may include an obstetrician prescribing methadone for a drug misuser presenting with opiate withdrawal in late pregnancy, an A&E doctor prescribing to a patient with serious concomitant physical or psychiatric illness where withdrawal is complicating the clinical problems, and when there is an acute hospital admission of somebody who is opiate-dependent. Indeed, in such circumstances it is vital that the doctor fulfil their responsibilities by ensuring adequate assessment and appropriate management that facilitates the retention of the patient in treatment.

1. Aims of assessment

1. To treat any emergency or acute problem.

2. Confirm patient is taking drugs (history, examination and urine analysis).

3. Assess degree of dependence.

4. Identify complications of drug misuse and assess risk behaviour.

5. Identify other medical, social and mental health problems.

6. Give advice on harm minimisation, including, if appropriate, access to sterile needles and syringes, testing for hepatitis, HIV and immunisation against hepatitis B.

7. Determine the patient's expectations of treatment and the degree of motivation to change.

8. Assess the most appropriate level of expertise required to manage the patient (this may alter over time), and refer/liaise appropriately (i.e. shared care, specialist or specialised generalist care) or other forms of psychosocial care where appropriate.

9. Determine the need for substitute medication – in the case of the generalist, this should be with advice from a specialist or specialised generalist, ideally through shared care structures.

10. Notify the patient to the local Regional Drug Misuse Database using the appropriate local reporting form.

11. In private practice establish that the patient is able to pay for treatment through legitimate means.

Introduction

Patients present, or are referred, for a variety of reasons. In some cases, an impending court case will precipitate presentation. The outcome for patients referred through the criminal justice system can be similar to that for patients who self-refer. Patients may consult a doctor for a medical problem without mentioning any drug use or misuse. By maintaining an empathic, non-judgemental attitude, the doctor may encourage appropriate disclosure.

Assessment should balance the needs of the patient with those of the medical practitioner. The doctor must ensure that an adequate assessment has been made before prescribing substitute opiates or other controlled drugs.

No doctor should feel pressurised into issuing substitute medication until he or she is satisfied that an appropriate assessment has been completed.

In most circumstances initial assessment may take more than one consultation.

When an assessment has been conducted, consideration needs to be given to the possibility that residential treatment, or other forms of psychosocial rehabilitation, is the treatment of choice. In such circumstances, further Community Care Assessment should be sought.

Irrespective of the drug of misuse with which the patient presents, the same fundamental aims of assessment apply.

The nature of the first consultation will depend upon whether or not the doctor is aware that the patient is seeking advice about a drug-related problem. If this is the first contact, it may be helpful to offer a longer appointment which allows enough time for a full diagnostic interview and physical examination. Concerned relatives or professionals already involved should be encouraged to attend with the patient. Doctors should have a significant role in health education regarding drug misuse, and will find value in giving accurate information to minimise the harm of more persistent drug taking and the risks of developing significant dependence.

2. Diagnosis of drug abuse

a) Drug history

The aim is to elicit as accurately as possible something about past and current drug-taking behaviour. It should cover the following areas:

> **i) Reason for presentation**
> - In crisis
> - Impending court case/in prison
> - Referred from court
> - On the recommendation of the court or a social worker
> - Want information and advice about the effects of the drug they are taking
> - Have had a recent health risk or have anxieties over their drug taking
> - Their behaviour is causing concern to others e.g. may have been brought along by a concerned parent, or friends
> - Suffering from mental illness
> - Pregnant
> - Want help with their drug misuse and motivated to change behaviour
> - Had enough! or usual source of drugs no longer available
> - Referred from another medical practitioner

ii) Past and current (last 4 weeks) drug use

- The age of starting drug misuse (including alcohol and nicotine)
- Types and quantities of drugs taken (including concomitant alcohol misuse)
- Frequency of misuse and routes of administration
- Experience of overdose
- Periods of abstinence? If yes, triggers for relapse?
- Symptoms experienced when unable to obtain their drugs?
- Cost of drug/alcohol misuse

iii) History of injecting and risk of HIV and hepatitis

- Past history
- Current usage and why patient changed to injecting
- Supply of needles and syringes
- Sharing habits, including lending and borrowing injection equipment/paraphernalia
- Does patient know how to inject safely?
- How does patient clean equipment?
- How does patient dispose of used equipment/'works'?
- Knowledge of HIV/Hep B and C issues and transmission
- Use of condoms
- Has patient ever thought of/tried other methods of use?

iv) Medical history

- Complications of drug use – abscesses, thrombosis, viral illnesses, chest problems
- Hepatitis B, C status if known
- HIV status if known
- Last cervical smear
- Last menstrual period
- Operations, accidents, head injury

v) Psychiatric history

- Psychiatric admissions/outpatient attendance
- Any overdoses (accidental or deliberate)?
- Any previous episodes of depression or psychosis? Treatment by GP with any psychotropic or analgesics at any time?

---

vi) Forensic history

- Past and present contact with the criminal justice system including probation/community service
- Past custodial sentences?
- Currently offending?
- Outstanding charges?

---

vii) Social history

- Family situation – especially children
- Employment situation
- Accommodation situation
- Financial situation, including debt

---

viii) Past contact with treatment services

- Previous efforts to reduce or stop taking drugs
- Contact with other doctors, social services, community services
- Previous rehabilitation admissions, how long they lasted and the cause of any relapses

---

ix) Other

- Drug and alcohol misuse in partner, spouse and other family members
- Impact of drug misuse on other aspects of the patient's life

---

b) Examination

i) Assessing motivation

Is the drug misuser motivated to stop or change their pattern of drug use or to make other changes in their life? Here you may need to encourage realism and what short-, intermediate- and long-term goals the patient seeks.

The drug misuser is not helped to make changes by being continuously rejected by treatment services, and every effort should be made to encourage motivation. Often, where there is resistance to change drug misuse itself, there is motivation to make changes in other parts of life e.g. personal relationships, accommodation and employment.

ii) Assessing general health

Medical

Physical examination is an important part of the assessment process, to assess the health of the drug user and to confirm the history (e.g. signs of drug misuse such as needle track marks, skin abscesses, and signs of withdrawal or intoxication) and to determine the presence of any complications of drug misuse.

Generally there is a greater prevalence of certain illnesses amongst the drug-misusing population, including viral hepatitis, bacterial endocarditis, HIV, tuberculosis, septicaemia, pneumonia, deep vein thrombosis, pulmonary emboli, abscesses and dental disease.

Injecting drug misuse carries the greatest risk of infection, particularly when equipment is shared or inadequately cleaned. Dirty and unhygienic injecting habits can result in local or systemic infections and poor injecting technique can cause venous or arterial thrombosis. Some drug misusers inject subcutaneously ('skin-popping') and some intramuscularly, but the most favoured route is intravenous, with the associated increased risk of overdose.

Complications of drug use

A: Drug related:	Side effects (e.g. constipation, hallucinations)
	Overdose (e.g. respiratory depression)
	Withdrawal (e.g. irritability, fits)

| B: Route specific: | Smoking (asthma) |
| | Injecting (abscesses, cellulitis) |

| C: Sharing needles, syringes and injection equipment: | Hepatitis B and C, HIV and other blood-borne viruses. |

| D: General: | Anaemia, poor nutrition, dental caries and erosion of dentine |

iii) Assessment of mental health

This is an essential part of the assessment process:

- Psychiatric problems sometimes co-exist with drug and alcohol misuse, in particular increased risk of suicide and self-harm.

- Drug of misuse often has a psychoactive component, e.g. can cause hallucinations (cocaine), depression or anxiety, either during use or as part of withdrawal.

It should include an examination of:

- General behaviour: e.g. restlessness, anxiety, irritability can be caused by either intoxication with stimulants or hallucinogens, or by withdrawal from opiates.

- Mood: depression can be caused by withdrawal from stimulants ('crash' of cocaine or amphetamine withdrawal) or by alcohol or sedative drugs. Assess the risk of self-harm.

- Delusions and hallucinations: common with stimulant and hallucinogens use.

- Confusional states

iv) Assessment of social and family situation

Assessment must include consideration of overall social, family responsibilities and housing stability and general welfare. Individuals with multiple social problems need to be linked into the appropriate local support networks. In some instances, Community Care Assessment will assist also to determine whether residential or day care services have a role to play.

c) Special investigations

i) Haematological investigations
- Haemoglobin
- Creatinine
- Liver function tests
- Hepatitis B
- Hepatitis C
- Test for HIV antibody

Before any test, full informed consent should be obtained from the patient.

ii) Urine assessment

Urine analysis should be regarded as an adjunct to the history and examination in confirming drug use, and should be obtained at the outset of prescribing and randomly throughout treatment. Results should always be interpreted in the light of clinical findings, as false negatives and positives can occur.

A urine test shows the range of drugs that are being used and, unless specially requested, results from laboratories are qualitative rather than quantitative. If the drug misuser is dependent, opiates persist in the urine for up to 24 hours (methadone up to 48 hours). Approximate drug detection times in urine are shown below in Table 1.

Ask the patient to produce a specimen on the premises. Usually about 5–10 ml, in a universal container, is sufficient. Though supervision of urine collection lessens the likelihood of introducing a substituted or contaminated sample, it is often impracticable to do and may be considered to be a breach of human dignity. Samples at body temperature are more likely to be from the patient. If there are doubts about the validity of the specimen offered this should be used as an opportunity to initiate a discussion with the patient about this concern. Routine urine samples are not suitable for medico-legal purposes.

Highly sensitive dipsticks for commonly misused substances are increasingly available, and can be especially valuable when instant validation is required as part of urgent clinical management.

If results do not correspond to the patient's history, repeat the urine toxicology test before taking any action, as laboratory errors can occur. If the urine test is negative and there is no evidence of withdrawal symptoms, the drug misuser is very unlikely to be physically dependent and should be reassessed in the light of this.

iii) Hair analysis

A single strand of hair can yield information covering a period of several weeks or months. Hair analysis is increasingly employed commercially in pre-employment screening for drug misuse. Hair analysis potentially has a place in the treatment of drug misuse, particularly in methadone treatment.[2]

3.   Reporting to the Regional Drug Misuse Databases

All doctors treating drug misusers for their problem drug misuse should provide information on a standard form to their local Regional Drug Misuse Database. Copies of the forms are available from the Database manager. There is a list of contact telephone numbers in these Guidelines.[3] Contact numbers are also given in the *British National Formulary*. Database managers can also provide detailed local analyses on request.

A report to the Drug Misuse Database should be made when a patient first presents with a drug problem or re-presents after a gap of six months or more.

All types of problem drug misuse should be reported e.g. opiate, benzodiazepine, stimulant.

The Drug Misuse Databases are the only national and local source of epidemiological data on people presenting to services for problem drug misuse, and as such provide valuable information to those working with, and those planning, services for drug misusers. Information on all drugs of misuse is obtained, but, because the data are anonymised, the databases cannot be used as a check on multiple prescribing for drug addicts.

---

[1] Wolff K., Welch S., Marsden J., Strang J., Farrell M., *Working group on identification and management of psychoactive substance use problems in primary health care settings*. WHO, 1997.
[2] McPhillips M., Strang J., Barnes T. 'Hair analysis. New laboratory ability to test for substance use'. *The British Journal of Psychiatry* 1998; **173**: 287–290.
[3] See Annex 19

Table 1:

Approximate duration of detectability of selected drugs in urine[1]

SUBSTANCE	DURATION OF DETECTABILITY
Amphetamines	48 hours
Methamphetamine	48 hours
Barbiturates	
short-acting	24 hours
intermediate-acting	48–72 hours
long-acting	7 days or more
Benzodiazepines	3 days (therapeutic dose)
ultra-short-acting (half-life 2 hours) (e.g. Midazolam)	12 hours
– short-acting (half-life 2–6 hours) (e.g. Triazolam)	24 hours
– intermediate-acting (half-life 6 24 hours)	
(e.g. Temazepam/Chlordiazepoxide)	40–80 hours
– long-acting (half-life 24 hours)	
(e.g. Diazepam/Nitrazepam)	7 days
Cocaine Metabolites	2–3 days
Methadone (maintenance dosing)	7–9 days (approximate)
Codeine/Morphine/Propoxyphene	
(Heroin is detected in urine as	48 hours
the metabolite morphine)	
Norpropoxyphene	6–48 hours
Cannabinoids (Marijuana)	
– single use	3 days
– moderate use (4 times per week)	4 days
– heavy use (daily)	10 days
– chronic heavy use	21–27 days
Methaqualone	7 days or more
Phencyclidine (PCP)	8 days (approximate)

CHAPTER 4
THE RESPONSIBILITIES AND PRINCIPLES OF PRESCRIBING FOR DRUG DEPENDENCE

This chapter will deal with the general principles of safe, evidence-based and effective prescribing. See Annex 13 for the technicalities of writing a prescription for controlled drugs.

Key chapter recommendations

> Prescribing should be seen as an enhancement to other psychological, social and medical interventions.

> As newer 'addiction' drug treatments are developed, clinicians are advised to request specialist advice to support the benefits of the pharmacological intervention they are either considering or being requested to prescribe.

> Keep good, clear, written or computerised records of prescribing.

> It is good practice for all new prescriptions to be taken initially under daily supervision for a minimum of three months – supervision should be undertaken at any stage during a prescription if considered appropriate.

> Methadone has to be clearly labelled and all bottles should have child-proof tops. The patient should be told that methadone and other prescribed drugs must be kept out of reach of children.

> Where the parent is opiate-dependent, and in receipt of a substitute drug prescription, their children should not be authorised to collect their medication from the pharmacy.

There are a number of drugs listed in these Clinical Guidelines, which are used outside the licensed indication. It is important to note that prescribing of licensed medications outside the recommendations of the product's licence alters (and generally increases) the doctor's professional responsibility.

The minimum responsibilities of the prescribing doctor

1. It is the responsibility of all doctors to provide care for general health needs and drug-related problems, whether or not the patient is ready to withdraw from drugs.

2. Medical practitioners should not prescribe substitute medication, such as methadone, in isolation. A multidisciplinary approach to drug treatment is essential.

3. Prescribing is the particular responsibility of the doctor signing the prescription. The responsibility cannot be delegated.

4. A doctor prescribing controlled drugs for the management of drug dependence should have an understanding of the basic pharmacology, toxicology and clinical indications for the use of the drug, dose regime and therapeutic monitoring strategy if they are to prescribe responsibly.

5. A full assessment of the patient, in conjunction with other professionals involved, should always be undertaken and treatment goals set.

6. The clinician has a responsibility to ensure that the patient receives the correct dose and that appropriate efforts are taken to ensure that the drug is used appropriately and not diverted onto the illegal market. Particular care must be taken with induction on to any substitute medication, especially where self-reporting of dosage is being relied upon.

7. Supervised consumption is recommended for new prescriptions for a minimum of three months, and should be relaxed only when the patient's compliance is assured. However, the need for supervised consumption should take into account the patient's social factors, such as employment and child care responsibilities. If supervised ingestion clashes with these and is still felt necessary, it must be made available at a time that allows the patient to attend without putting their job or families at risk.

8. The prescribing doctor should liaise regularly with the dispensing pharmacist about the specific patient and the prescribing regime.

9. No more than one week's drugs should be dispensed at one time, except in exceptional circumstances.

10. Clinical reviews should be undertaken regularly, at least every three months, particularly in patients whose drug use remains unstable.

11. The patient should be told that methadone and other prescribed drugs must be kept out of reach of children.

12. Thorough, clearly written or computer records of prescribing should be kept.

Prescribing

1.   The responsibility of prescribing

Prescribing is the particular responsibility of the doctor signing the prescription. The responsibility cannot be delegated.

A decision to prescribe, what and how much to prescribe will depend upon:

i)   the overall treatment plan for the individual patient;

ii)   these Clinical Guidelines;

iii)   locally agreed protocols;

iv)   the doctor's experience and level of training;

v)   discussion with other members of a multidisciplinary team;

vi)   advice, where necessary, from a specialist in drug misuse.

In the context of prescribing, it is important to note that the *British National Formulary* (BNF) is a key reference. The dosages stated in these Clinical Guidelines and in the BNF are intended for general guidance and represent (unless otherwise stated) the range of dosages that are generally regarded as being suitable for prescribing in the context of treating adults who have become dependent.

2.   Deciding whether to prescribe

Before deciding whether to prescribe, the doctor should be clear as to what the functions of a prescription are. A prescription can:

i)   reduce or prevent withdrawal symptoms;

ii)   offer an opportunity to stabilise drug intake and lifestyle whilst breaking with previous illicit drug use and associated unhealthy behaviours;

iii)   promote a process of change in drug taking and risk behaviour;

iv)   help to maintain contact and offer an opportunity to work with the patient.

A prescription for substitute drugs should only be considered if:

i)   the drug/s is/are being taken on a regular basis – particularly for daily misuse;

ii)   there is convincing evidence of current dependence (including objective signs of withdrawal symptoms wherever possible);

iii)   the patient is motivated to change at least some aspects of their drug use;

iv)   the assessment (history, urine toxicology, drug diary) clearly substantiates the need for treatment;

v)   the doctor is satisfied that the patient will co-operate and demonstrate adequate compliance with the prescribing regime.

3.   Setting goals[1]

Before prescribing substitute drugs the doctor should establish:

i)   what changes the patient wishes to make in the way he or she uses drugs;

ii)   what lifestyle changes the patient wants to make;

iii)   how a prescription might help the patient to achieve these changes.

In the light of the changes that the drug misuser would like to make; set mutually agreed and realistic goals to be achieved within 4 to 12 weeks of starting the prescription. For example:

- to begin to tackle other problem areas e.g. legal, financial, accommodation and relationship problems;
- to reduce or stop using illicit drugs;
- to review alcohol consumption;
- to reduce frequency of injecting;
- to attend appointments on time.

Goals should be recorded and reviewed regularly throughout the period of treatment.

---

[1] (From) *Managing drug users in general practice*. 2nd edition. Lothian Health Board, 1996.

4. Ending a failing treatment

The decision to end a failing treatment should not be taken lightly, and should ideally be part of a treatment plan agreed with the patient. However, if a patient receiving treatment for drug misuse fails to comply with that treatment, and consistently fails to make progress towards agreed and reasonable goals, the doctor may have to consider ending that particular treatment.

It may be possible to agree with the patient some modified goals which require very little treatment input, or it may be necessary to acknowledge that nothing currently is being achieved and treatment contact will cease.

Due notice should be given of a reduction regime. Suggestions for referral for further assessment with local specialist services, to consider other treatment options and arrangements, will mean the patient still has access to general medical care.

When a patient has successfully finished the treatment offered by a specific agency the individual's general practitioner should be informed. Clinicians and the agencies they work with should carry out some kind of formal clinical audit of their discharged patients. Where possible, some objective evaluation of the treatment effectiveness of the agency should be incorporated.

5. The choice of drug

a) What to prescribe

- It is usually better to use longer-acting opiate agonists (e.g. methadone) in opiate dependence and long-acting benzodiazepines (e.g. diazepam or chlordiazepoxide) in benzodiazepine dependence, rather than shorter-acting drugs or preparations.

- Whilst it may be easier initially to titrate dose against effect, it is harder to maintain stability on shorter-acting drugs.

- There are satisfactory non-opiate treatments (e.g. lofexidine), which are useful in the treatment of withdrawal.

- Though there is a very limited place for the prescribing of injectable formulations by specialists, prescribing should generally aim to minimise injecting.

b) Initiating prescribing

- The aim is to prescribe a dose of a substitute drug that will prevent withdrawal symptoms and reduce or eliminate non-prescribed drug use.

- Dose consumption should usually be supervised by either the doctor, a nurse or community pharmacist. In the rare event that such initial doses are to be taken unsupervised, the dose should be set so as to minimise the risk of diversion onto the black market or unsolicited use.

- Titrate the calculated dose against any continuing withdrawal symptoms.

- Review the treatment regimen regularly enough to ensure compliance.

c) The route of administration

- Oral medication should be in a non-injectable form, i.e. liquid mixture.

- Tablet forms that are likely to be crushed and inappropriately injected should not be prescribed e.g. methadone tablets or other tableted opiates.

d) Prescribing injectable drugs

There is a small section of the treatment population who, despite continued treatment with oral preparations, fail to make adequate progress and continue to be involved in high levels of injecting drug misuse and other risk-taking behaviour. These patients may benefit from specialist assessment: in some instances, clinical benefit can be improved by correcting sub-optimum dosing, although for others specialists could decide to initiate a prescription for a drug taken by injection.

6. Record keeping

There should be clear and concise notes, properly signed, named and dated. A separate structured sheet for recording prescribing may be helpful. A patient-held record, countersigned by those involved in care, can be a useful adjunct to treatment.

Other doctors who may see the patient should be informed of current treatment. The patient should ideally be seen on each occasion by the prescribing doctor or an informed colleague.

7. Dispensing

The basic arrangements for effective dispensing are as follows:

- Wherever possible, liaise with the dispensing pharmacist about the specific patient and the prescribing regimen.[2] Inform the pharmacist if the prescriber has a special prescribing licence or a handwriting dispensation.

---

[2] *Report of the Working Party on Pharmaceutical Services for Drug Misusers*. London: The Royal Pharmaceutical Society of Great Britain, 1998. This report recommends that prescribers should contact a pharmacist, prior to issuing a new prescription, in order to discuss the client's treatment and other practicalities (2.4.2).

■ As a general principle, substitute drugs should be dispensed on a daily basis.

■ For some patients, supervised consumption should be arranged with the most appropriate health professional, e.g. clinic nurse, community pharmacist.

■ If the patient is clearly making satisfactory progress on a daily dispensing regimen, the dispensing intervals can be reduced gradually to thrice weekly, then twice weekly, etc.

■ In most circumstances, no more than a week's total dose should be dispensed at one time, except for holidays and special arrangements.

■ Unless there are compelling reasons, such as immobility, the patient whose name appears on the prescription should collect the medication themselves from the pharmacist.

8. Issues for special vigilance

To minimise further the risk of inappropriate diversion onto the illicit drugs market, doctors and professionals in multidisciplinary teams must have regard for the security of drugs, prescription pads and headed notepaper, and take sensible precautions to avoid the risk of theft of items such as these. Additional suggestions are listed in the *British National Formulary* in the section dealing with Controlled Drugs.

CHAPTER 5
THE MANAGEMENT OF DEPENDENCE AND WITHDRAWAL

Key chapter recommendations

> For all reduction regimes, prior dose assessment, a period of stabilisation with a substitute drug (which may be over several days or weeks), supervised ingestion (at least in the initial period) and a regular review of treatment aims should be undertaken.

> Doctors need to understand that the first two weeks of treatment with methadone is associated with a substantially increased risk of overdose mortality. Starting a prescription requires careful assessment for evidence of opiate dependence, withdrawal and tolerance, and the use of confirmatory tests such as urine screening. Furthermore, good knowledge of the pharmacology and toxicology of the drugs prescribed and a careful induction regimen is critical. This should ensure that, in the early phase, dosages of the drug are not prescribed that could result in a fatal overdose, either alone or in combination with other prescribed or non-prescribed drugs.

Introduction

For presentational reasons, a distinction is drawn between withdrawal, detoxification (rapid and gradual) and maintenance, as well as their associated prescribing patterns. In practice, however, these categories overlap, and the reader is cautioned against expecting such clear distinctions in clinical practice.

While there are currently only a limited number of treatments available to assist in keeping people free of drugs, there is a considerable interest in research on possible blocking drugs and new anti-craving agents that might assist in this process. One of the challenges for the future is to find ways to integrate new drug treatment approaches with new psychological approaches that are aimed at helping the individual to maintain whatever health-conferring behavioural change they achieve.

Overall, this chapter covers issues of prescribing in the context of the management of drug dependence. It summarises the best available evidence on a range of clinical approaches. It emphasises the key points raised in the previous chapter and encourages clinicians to exercise caution in prescribing practice by:

– adhering to the use of medications that have been licensed by the Medicines Control Agency (MCA) for the treatment of drug dependence, except in exceptional circumstances.

– prescribing medications in a manner that ensures they are dispensed safely (e.g. on a daily basis) and consumed by the named patient himself/herself (e.g. under supervision).

– ensuring that a capacity to monitor progress and review overall treatment goals is integral to the decision to prescribe and the subsequent provision of care.

1. Withdrawal/detoxification

For some individuals, general support, understanding of the symptomatology and encouragement may suffice. Symptomatic relief of withdrawal symptoms can sometimes be achieved without substitute medication.

Some people can withdraw without the aid of a prescription. Studies of self-recovery by drug users show that shifts in identity and lifestyle, together with changes in an individual's environment, are important in the pathway out of addiction.[1,2,3] For others, however, a history of serious withdrawal complications (e.g. benzodiazepine or alcohol withdrawal-induced epileptic fits), or a lack of social support or other problems, may make substitute prescribing necessary. It is best to assume that any drug that has been heavily consumed over a significant period of time may have a withdrawal-symptom profile associated with it. Such an approach will assist drug misusers in their preparation to withdraw from cocaine, amphetamines and also cannabis. Withdrawal symptoms will differ depending on the pharmacological profile of the drug misuser. Some drugs with short half-lives will give rise to withdrawal symptoms at an earlier phase: the symptoms will also peak, and be cleared, quicker.

The severity of withdrawal symptoms is not clearly or directly related to the quantity of drugs previously consumed. When assessing withdrawal, for the purpose of dose titration, it is better to place greater weight on observable signs rather than subjective symptoms.

Detoxification refers to the withdrawal over a short period from an opioid or sedative/hypnotic drug by the use of the same drug, or a similar drug, in decreasing doses. The process can be assisted by the temporary prescription of other drugs to reduce withdrawal symptoms.

2. Opiates

Withdrawal from opiates is associated with a specific withdrawal syndrome.

- ■ Untreated heroin withdrawal typically reaches its peak 36–72 hours after the last dose and symptoms will have subsided substantially after 5 days.

[1] Biemacki P., *Pathways from Heroin Addiction: recovery without treatment*. Philadelphi: Temple University Press, 1986.
[2] Waldorf D., 'Natural recovery from opiate addiction: some social-psychological processes of untreated recovery.' *Journal of Drug Issues* 1983; **13**: 237–280.
[3] Robins L., *The Vietnam Drug User Returns*. Washington D.C.: US Government Printing Office, 1973.

■ Untreated methadone withdrawal typically reaches its peak between 4 to 6 days and symptoms do not substantially subside for 10 to 12 days.

a) Symptoms and signs of opiate withdrawal

1) Sweating
2) Lachrymation and rhinorrhea*
3) Yawning*
4) Feeling hot and cold*
5) Anorexia and abdominal cramps*
6) Nausea, vomiting and diarrhoea*
7) Tremor
8) Insomnia and restlessness*
9) Generalised aches and pains*
10) Tachycardia, hypertension*
11) Gooseflesh
12) Dilated pupils
13) Increased bowel sounds

Those asterisked in the above list comprise the Opiate Withdrawal Scale (OWS) for which psychometric properties have been published[4] and which is extensively used in the UK to quantify the severity of the withdrawal syndrome.

b) Treatment of the withdrawal syndrome with substitute opiates

i) Methadone

Detoxification with methadone can be undertaken under a number of different regimens in the short and long term. Dose regimens are given later in this chapter.

The medication of choice is Methadone mixture BNF 1mg/ml.
It is licensed for the treatment of opiate dependence.

– it is longer acting (typically 24 – 48 hours) making stability from daily dosing easier to achieve;
– it is straightforward to titrate in order to achieve the correct dose;
– it is less likely to be diverted than shorter-acting drugs;
– it is less likely to be injected;
– its clinical effectiveness is supported by research.

True intolerance to methadone is very unusual. If the patient is clearly intolerant, (e.g. it induces vomiting, or, very rarely, an allergic reaction), dihydrocodeine can be used.

---

[4] Gossop M., Darke S., Griffiths P., Hando J., Powis B., Hall W., Strang J., 'The Severity of Dependence Scale. psychometric properties of the SDS in English and Australian samples of heroin, cocaine and amphetamine users.' *Addiction* 1995; **90**: 607–614.

Intolerance to liquid methadone is not an indication for injectable methadone.

Dose reduction, using methadone, can take place at any pace depending on the results of the assessment and treatment plan. The most rapid regime can be carried out by incremental cuts in dose over 7–21 days; slower regimes may take several months to complete. The general principle being that at higher dose levels the greater the reduction possible, as it represents a smaller percentage of the total. As the dose falls, reduction should be more gradual. Dose reductions can occur at any time interval, e.g. daily, alternate days, weekly.

It may be necessary to hold the reduction steady at a given dose over a few days to decrease the patient's anxiety and increase their sense of control. Delays in the rate of reduction should be accompanied by psychological support.

ii) Codeine-based drugs

Not licensed for use for the treatment of drug dependence.

Though there is little in the published literature, some experienced practitioners use codeine-based substitute drugs, including dihydrocodeine, either as the principle drug in treating opiate withdrawal (for patients already stabilised on a prescription of dihydrocodeine) or as an adjunct to a methadone withdrawal programme, where it may be used to counter withdrawal symptoms towards the end of a reducing methadone regime, usually when the methadone dose reaches around 15mg.[5] However, the product licence for dihydrocodeine does not include the treatment of opiate dependence, and there is concern amongst practitioners about its widespread use.[6] Repeated tablet-taking throughout the day (necessary due to the drug's short half-life) may reinforce patterns of drug-taking behaviour and prohibit change. Those with severe opiate dependence may require large quantities of tablets, which may give rise to concerns over diversion.

iii) Buprenorphine

Licensed for the treatment of drug dependence.

This drug binds to morphine receptors, and has an effective duration of at least 24 hours. It is now available as an 8mg (eight) sublingual tablet, and can be taken daily.[7] In well-controlled studies it has been reported to be equivalent to 30mg of methadone. It is reported to have low euphoric effects at higher doses.[8] There is interest in its use as an alternative to methadone maintenance and also in the management of opiate withdrawal as its mixed agonist antagonist properties make it a potentially good agent for the management of opiate withdrawal. It is also reported to have lower overdose potential, however further research is required before detailed recommendations can be made. In the late 1980s, a wave of buprenorphine misuse in the form of injecting was reported in several parts of the UK, especially Glasgow. To a lesser extent, the North of England saw an increase in buprenorphine abuse in the mid-eighties, which was associated with injecting.[9]

---

[5] Macleod J., Whittaker A., Robertson J.R., 'Changes in opiate treatment during attendance at a community drug service – findings from a clinical audit.' *Drug and Alcohol Review* 1998; **17**: 19–25.

[6] Swadi H., Wells B., Power R., 'Misuse of dihydrocodeine tartrate (DF 118) among opiate addicts.' *British Medical Journal* 1990; **300**: 1313.

[7] Johnson R., Eissenberg T., Stitzer M., Strain E., Liebson I., Bigelow G., 'Buprenorphine treatment of opioid dependence: clinical trial of daily versus alternate-day dosing.' *Drug and Alcohol Dependence* 1995; **40**: 27–35.

[8] Walsh S.L., Preston K.L., Stitzer M.L., Cone E.J., Bigelow G.E., 'Clinical pharmacology of buprenorphine: ceiling effects at high doses.' *Clinical Pharmacology and Therapeutics* 1994; **55**: 569–580.

[9] Sakol M.S., Stark C., Sykes R., 'Buprenorphine and temazepam abuse by drug takers in Glasgow – an increase.' *British Journal of Addiction* 1989; **84**: 439–41.

It is recommended that buprenorphine should be initiated by a specialist practitioner, and safeguards such as daily dispensing, with supervised consumption, should be inherent to any well-delivered buprenorphine substitution programme. The ready solubility and injectability of this substance makes it a substance that requires longer term supervised dispensing but this could be reviewed when a product that combines buprenorphine and naloxone becomes available in the future.[10] Given the limited experience in the UK with this new form of buprenorphine, it is recommended that thorough evaluation be conducted to explore the possible benefits and drawbacks that may be conferred by this new pharmacological option.

c) Treatment of the withdrawal syndrome with non-opiate drugs

There are now satisfactory non-opiate treatments (such as lofexidine) for opiate withdrawal. These are:

- effective in alleviating opiate-withdrawal symptoms;
- not liable to, or less open to, misuse by the patient;
- less likely to be diverted on to the black market.

i) Lofexidine

Licensed for the management of symptoms of opiate withdrawal.

Lofexidine is now fully licensed in the UK for the management of the symptoms of opiate withdrawal. It is a useful non-opiate treatment for opiate addiction. Lofexidine hydrochloride is similar in action to clonidine, but causes much less hypotension. It can be used with supervision in inpatient, residential and community settings. There is evidence to suggest that it is equally as efficacious as methadone in withdrawal.[11, 12, 13] Lofexidine has a role in the treatment of opiate-dependent individuals seeking abstinence and whose drug use is already well controlled. Some experienced doctors use lofexidine prior to and during initial assessment, to control symptoms of opiate withdrawal and enable a full assessment to take place. It is also sometimes useful to control symptoms when a patient claims to have lost a prescription for methadone, instead of reissuing the methadone prescription or refusing to prescribe.

ii) Clonidine

Not licensed for the treatment of opiate withdrawal symptoms.

Clonidine has also been used in the management of opiate withdrawal. It is useful as a non-opiate treatment for opiate withdrawal. Clonidine was originally developed for the management of high blood pressure and has a substantial hypotensive effect. For this reason there is a need to monitor blood pressure and to modify or withdraw the treatment if symptomatic hypotension occurs.

---

[10] Reynaud M., Petit G., Potard D., Courty P., 'Six deaths linked to concomitant use of buprenorphine and benzodiazepines.' *Addiction* 1998; **93**: 1385–1392.
[11] Bearn J., Gossop M., Strang J., 'Randomised double-blind comparison of lofexidine and methadone in the in-patient treatment of opiate withdrawal.' *Drug and Alcohol Dependence* 1996; **43**: 87–91.
[12] Brown A.S., Fleming P.M., 'A naturalistic study of home detoxification from opiates using lofexidine.' *Journal of Psychopharmacology* 1998; **12**: 93–96.
[13] Carnwath T., Hardman J., 'Randomised double-blind comparison of lofexidine and clonidine in the out-patient treatment of opiate withdrawal.' *Drug and Alcohol Dependence* 1998; **50**: 251–254.

iii) Naltrexone

Not currently licensed for the purposes of detoxification, but licensed only as an adjunct to prevent relapse in detoxified, formerly opioid-dependent, patients who have remained opioid free for at least 7–10 days.

Naltrexone blocks opiate effects for up to 72 hours, hence it needs to be ingested only three times per week. 'Rapid' detoxification over 5 to 7 days utilising naltrexone to precipitate withdrawal symptoms is now available in some specialist centres.[14] This technique should be carried out by specialists with inpatient facilities. The effectiveness and safety of rapid anaesthetic-antagonist detoxification as a treatment method has not yet been established.

iv) Other drugs

There is a range of drugs (some available over the counter) which can be used to reduce the physical effects of withdrawal (itching/ insomnia/ anxiety/ diarrhoea/ pains).

For example:

Loperamide hydrochloride (Imodium), Co-Phenotrope (Lomotil) – use in standard doses for the treatment of diarrhoea.

Metoclopramide hydrochloride – use to treat nausea and vomiting, may also be useful for treatment of stomach cramps.

Non-steroidal anti-inflammatory drugs (NSAIDS) – use to alleviate muscular pains and headaches.

3.   Benzodiazepines

Not licensed for the management of benzodiazepine dependence, licensed for short-term use for the management of insomnia and anxiety and benzodiazepine withdrawal.

These drugs have their own addictive potential and are often taken in combination with opiates. Up to 90 per cent of attenders at drug misuse treatment centres reported use of benzodiazepines in a one-year period,[15] and 49 per cent had injected them.[16]

Sudden cessation in the use of benzodiazepines can lead to a recognised withdrawal state.[17,18]

---

[14] Brewer C., 'On the specific effectiveness, and under-valuing, of pharmacological treatments for addiction: a comparison of methadone, naltrexone and disulfiram with psychosocial interventions.' *Addiction Research* 1996; **3**: 297–313.

[15] Perera K.M., Tulley M., Jenner F.A., 'The use of benzodiazepines among drug addicts.' *British Journal of Addiction* 1987; **82**: 511–515.

[16] Strang J., Griffiths P., Abbey J., Gossop M., 'Survey of use of injected benzodiazepines among drug users in Britain.' *British Medical Journal* 1994; **308**: 1082

[17] Noyes R., Garvey M.J., Cook B.L., Perry P.J., 'Benzodiazepine withdrawal: a review of the evidence.' *Journal of Clinical Psychiatry* 1988; **49**: 382–9.

[18] Seivewright N., Dougal W., 'Withdrawal symptoms from high dose benzodiazepines in polydrug users.' *Drug and Alcohol Dependence* 1993; **32**: 15–23.

a) Withdrawal syndrome associated with benzodiazepine use

Anxiety symptoms:

> anxiety
>
> sweating
>
> insomnia
>
> headache
>
> tremor
>
> nausea

Disordered perceptions:

> feelings of unreality
>
> abnormal body sensations
>
> abnormal sensation of movement
>
> hypersensitivity to stimuli

Major complications:

> psychosis
>
> epileptic seizures[19]

b) Prescribing

Withdrawal prescribing should only be initiated where there is clear evidence of benzodiazepine dependency from the patient's history and urine examination. Longer-term use of benzodiazepines should adhere to the general principles of management, including clear indications of benzodiazepine dependence, clear treatment goals and milestones, regular review and methods to prevent diversion.[20] There is no evidence to suggest that long-term substitute prescribing of benzodiazepines reduces the harm associated with benzodiazepine use and there is increasing evidence that long-term prescribing of more than 30mgs per day may cause harm. Doctors should be reluctant to initiate maintenance prescribing of substitute benzodiazepines and should gradually reduce the doses of those already on a maintenance script for more than 30mgs per day.

If the patient is also receiving a long-term prescription of methadone for concomitant opiate dependency, the methadone dose should be kept stable throughout the benzodiazepine reduction period. Concurrent detoxification of both drugs is not recommended in a community setting.

A short course lasting only a few days may help alleviate anxiety and insomnia. However, doctors should guard against longer prescribing regimens that might induce addiction and inadvertently become maintenance prescribing.

---

[19] Busto U., Sellers E.M., Naranjo C.A., Cappell H., Sanchez-Craig M., Sykora K., 'Withdrawal reaction after long-term therapeutic use of benzodiazepines.' *New England Journal of Medicine* 1986; **315**: 854–859.
[20] Landry M.J., Smith D.E., McDuff D.R., Baughman O.L., 'Benzodiazepine dependence and withdrawal: identification and medical management.' *Journal of the American Board of Family Practitioners* 1992; **5**: 167–75.

---

4. Stimulants

A number of different compounds have been used in an attempt to reduce the symptoms of withdrawal and craving in stimulant users.[21]

a) General measures

General principles of management, such as giving preventive advice about safer injecting practice, must be applied. Psychiatric complications need to be treated on a symptomatic basis. Studies have found that an abstinence-based psychosocial treatment approach, linking counselling and social support, had the greatest impact on cocaine misuse.[22, 23]

Where a patient exhibits persistent anxiety and agitation, the clinician should attempt to focus on stress-reduction procedures. Patients who display persistent and severe psychotic symptoms require admission and treatment in a psychiatric unit. Other stimulant users who are chaotic may benefit from a period of inpatient assessment with support.

Complementary therapies, such as acupuncture, are being more widely used for cocaine misuse, although there is only limited evidence to support their effectiveness. Such interventions in some settings are clearly capable of attracting a hard to reach population into treatment and should be explored specifically for this purpose.

b) Antidepressants

Antidepressants, such as fluoxetine, can be effective in the management of major depressive episodes associated with stimulant use. Care should be taken if selective serotonin re-uptake inhibitors are prescribed whilst cocaine or amphetamine continue to be taken, as toxic reactions have been described.[24]

c) Substitute prescribing

There is no indication for the prescription of cocaine or methylamphetamine in the treatment of stimulant withdrawal, and it is not recommended that other stimulants, such as methylphenidate or phentermine, are prescribed.

There may be a limited place for the prescription of dexamphetamine sulphate 5mg (five) in the treatment of amphetamine misuse. There is evidence that such treatment is being undertaken quite

[21] Seivewright N.. McMahon C., 'Misuse of amphetamine and related drugs,' *Advances in Psychiatric Treatment* 1996; **2**: 211–218.

[22] Donmall M., Seivewright N., Douglas J., Draycott T., Millar T., 'National cocaine treatment study: the effectiveness of treatments offered to cocaine/crack users. A report to the Task Force,' London: Department of Health, 1995.

[23] Carroll K.M., Rounsaville B.J., Nich C., Gordon L., Gawin F., 'Integrating psychotherapy and pharmacotherapy for cocaine dependence: results from a randomized clinical trial'. *NIDA Res Monograph* 1995; **150**: 19–35.

[24] Barrett J., Meehan O., Fahy T., 'SSRI and sympathominetic interaction.' *British Journal of Psychiatry* 1996; **168**: 253.

widely in England and Wales[25] and there are a number of reports of its use from practitioners.[26, 27] However, to date there is only limited evidence to prove its effectiveness.[28]

Dexamphetamine prescribing should only be initiated by specialists and specialised generalists with adequate experience in this technique. Where shared care schemes are set up, arrangements should be clearly delineated between the specialist and the patient's general practitioner. The aim is not to give an equivalent dose to that used illegally but to minimise withdrawal symptoms and craving.

For those patients stabilised on a prescription of dexamphetamine, reduction can take place fairly rapidly. Withdrawal may be associated with significant depression: the patient's mood should be monitored and the risk of suicide assessed.

Dexamphetamine prescribing

Not licensed for the treatment of drug dependence.

Experienced practitioners limit dexamphetamine prescribing to the following cases:

- primary amphetamine users
- injecting users
- heavy, dependent use for more than three months, i.e. more than 1g (one) daily or on more than three days a week
- evidence of escalating use and increasing tolerance and craving

It is important that they are not prescribed in the following cases:

- polydrug use
- history of mental illness
- hypotension or heart disease
- pregnancy

There is no research to guide practitioners. The risk of paranoid symptoms should deter the use of high doses. Doses are usually given once a day in the morning. Daily dispensing is recommended. Avoid long-term prescribing, a strict time limit is preferable.

Injecting behaviour, illicit drug use, mental state, blood pressure, weight and urine, should all be monitored regularly.

If there is no progress towards any of the goals of treatment the prescription should be reviewed and stopped if necessary.

There is as yet no international consensus or endorsement of this practice.

---

[25] Strang J., Sheridan J., 'Prescribing amphetamines to drug misusers: data from the 1995 national survey of community pharmacies in England and Wales.' *Addiction* 1997; **92**: 833–838.

[26] Myles J., 'Treatment of Amphetamine Misuse in The United Kingdom', in *Amphetamine Misuse, International Perspectives on current Trends*, Klee H. (ed). Amsterdam: Harwood Academic Press, 1996.

[27] Fleming P.M., Roberts D., 'Is the prescription of amphetamine justified as a harm reduction measure?' *Journal of the Royal Society of Health* 1994; **114**: 127–131.

[28] Mattick R.P., Darke S., 'Drug replacement treatments. is amphetamine substitution a horse of a different colour?' *Drug and Alcohol Review* 1995; **14**: 398–394.

CHAPTER 6
DOSE REDUCTION REGIMENS

Key chapter recommendations

It is important to tailor the treatment needs to those of the individual needs of the presenting patient, especially where substitute treatment for dependence is concerned.

A dose reduction intervention should be shaped by a realistic appraisal of jointly agreed treatment goals and outcomes between the patient, the doctor and other members involved in the patient's care.

Treatment aims and goals should be adjusted accordingly depending on the patient's progress.

Methadone maintenance treatment, incorporating psychosocial interventions, can enable patients to achieve stability, reduce their drug misuse and criminal activity, and improve health. For these reasons such treatment should form an important part of drug misuse services.

There is now a choice of substances available for use in opiate maintenance prescribing. There is a need to monitor research progress in this field and to adjust future treatments in the light of new treatment evaluations.

1. Methadone mix BNF 1mg/ml

Licensed as an adjunct in treatment of opioid dependence.

a) Commencement dose

Initial doses of methadone should take into account the potential for opiate toxicity. This should include consideration of the assessment of the patient's opiate tolerance based on a history of the quantity, frequency and route of administration of opioids, use of other drugs such as benzodiazepines and alcohol, and also the long half-life of methadone.

The commencement dose should aim to achieve an effective level of comfort, both physical and psychological, while minimising the likelihood of overdose.

Inappropriate dosing can result in overdosing in the first few days: as cumulative toxicity develops to methadone, this can lead to death. Deaths have occurred following the commencement of a daily dose of 40mg methadone.

In general, the initial daily dose will be in the range of 10–40mg. If neuroadaptation (i.e. tolerance to opiates) is present then the usual daily dose is 25–40mg. If tolerance is low, or uncertain, then 10–20mg is more appropriate. Care is needed in starting a dose greater than 30mg because of the risk of overdose. If a low starting dose of 10mg is used, supervision after a few hours and further small doses can be given depending on the severity of the withdrawal symptoms.

In cases where dose assessment is undertaken, the patient should be re-assessed about 4 hours after the administration of an initial dose.

With heavily dependent users, i.e. those who are neuroadapted or tolerant, a first dose can be up to 40mg but it is unwise to exceed this dose. A second dose may follow after at least 4 hours and may be up to 30mg depending on the persisting severity of withdrawal. It is important that consideration is given to the cumulative effects of administering such a long-acting drug as methadone.

Severity of withdrawal	Additional dosage
Mild	No methadone
Moderate (muscle aches and pains, pupil dilatation, nausea, yawning)	5–10mg
Severe (vomiting, piloerection, tachycardia, elevated BP)	20–30mg

A supplementary dose should only be considered where there is evidence of persistent opioid withdrawal. These cases need to be assessed by an experienced medical practitioner.

b) Stabilisation dose

i) First seven days

If managing the opiate addict as an out-patient, it is recommended that patients attend daily during the first few days in order that their dose can be titrated against withdrawal symptoms and for assessment by the prescribing medical practitioner. Where doses need to be increased during the first seven days, the increment should be no more than 5mg to 10mg on one day. In any event, a total weekly increase should not usually exceed 30mg above the starting day's dose. Steady state plasma levels should be reached five days after the last dose increase.

ii) Subsequent stabilisation period

It is recommended that subsequent increases do not exceed 10mg per week up to a total of between 60 and 120mg. Stabilisation is usually complete by the end of the sixth week of methadone treatment, but this may take longer in some individuals.

It is critically important to provide adequate information regarding the recognition of methadone toxicity and management to patients and accompanying carers (with consent).

iii) Slow reduction regimes

After a period of stabilisation in which the patient should be encouraged to abstain completely from heroin, the daily dose can be reduced by 5mg to 10mg every week or fortnight until a stable dose is reached and the drug misuser continues to abstain from illegal drug use.

- In a four-month detoxification regime the dose would be reduced by 5mg every fortnight.
- In a six-month detoxification regime the dose would be reduced by 10mg every fortnight.

c) Drug reduction regimes

After a patient has become stabilised on the prescription, and has made other changes in lifestyle, it may be appropriate to set up a formal drug reduction regimen. In reality, patient compliance with a drug reduction regimen will only be maintained if patient and doctor both agree that reduction is desirable. There is usually very little clinical improvement when a reduction regimen is carried out against the wishes of the patient. Hence, if the patient is not going to be fully compliant, it is best to continue with the existing, stable regimen. The following issues should be considered:

i)   Stability on a substitute prescription offers the opportunity to discover and address those issues that have led to drug misuse. It may take months, or even years, for a drug misuser to reach a stage where a reduction in their prescribed drugs can be considered.

ii)   Many patients, despite requesting detoxification, are more suitable for maintenance treatment. The treatment options should be sensitively explored with the patient, and the overall goal should be to maximise the patient's potential health gain.

iii)   Undertaking a regular clinical review, on at least a three-monthly basis, of all long-term patients, will ensure that the potential goal of abstinence can always be re-considered. Better co-ordination of local services might enable substitute drug-maintained patients to become drug free.

2. Other pharmacotherapies

a) Lofexidine community detoxification

Licensed for the management of symptoms of opioid withdrawal.

The treatment course is between 7–10 days. It is probably most likely to be successful for patients with an average daily heroin use (up to 1gm per day or 50mg methadone equivalent), non polydrug users and those with shorter drug and treatment histories.

Reported side effects are a dry mouth and mild drowsiness. Sedation is increased with concomitant use of alcohol or central nervous system depressants. Overdose can result in hypotension, bradycardia, sedation and coma. Use with caution in patients with cardiac disease, cerebro-vascular accidents, and chronic renal failure. The safety in pregnant and breastfeeding women has not been established.

Before commencing a patient on lofexidine it is advisable to obtain a baseline blood pressure (BP) reading and then measure the BP over the first 2–3 days. Lofexidine should be discontinued if the blood pressure drops significantly. Patients sometimes complain of a metallic taste in their mouth and that their urine smells of yeast.

The patient should be seen daily in the early stages of treatment to check for withdrawal symptoms, for blood pressure monitoring and to provide general encouragement. Additional short-term medication for symptoms such as stomach cramps and diarrhoea may be required.

The patient should be advised to take at least part of their dose at bedtime to offset insomnia associated with opiate withdrawal.

b) Lofexidine detoxification regime

One tablet = 200 microgram

Initially 200 micrograms twice a day, increased daily as necessary, to control withdrawal, in steps of 200–400 micrograms daily to a maximum of 2.4mg. Recommended duration of treatment 7–10 days. Withdraw gradually over 2–4 days (or longer).

This regime may need to be altered in the light of withdrawal symptoms, with higher doses needed by some patients at the early stages of opiate withdrawal.

If lofexidine is used in the assessment stage, a dose of 200–400 micrograms (1–2 tablets) two to three times a day for 3–4 days is usually sufficient.

c) Dihydrocodeine

Not licensed for the management of drug dependence.

As with some of the other detoxification agents, there is some interest in the use of this and other opiates in the treatment of opiate dependence. Some practitioners take the view that dihydrocodeine can be useful to reduce the severity of withdrawal symptoms, as part of a reducing methadone regime, by switching to dihydrocodeine for the final part of the detoxification, usually when the methadone dose reaches around 15mg.

This is because dihydrocodeine is:

- a shorter acting drug with less severe withdrawal symptoms;

- a relatively weak opiate (30mg dihydrocodeine = 3mg methadone);

- easier to reduce slowly without practical difficulties, particularly if the 10mg per 5ml liquid formulation is used.

Some practitioners use up to 50 tablets a day for maintenance and gradual detoxification purposes. There are differing views about the value of different preparations, but the longer acting preparations (e.g. modified release dihydrocodeine tartrate 60mg – DHC Continus) are more easily supervised.

Many doctors see people who have become addicted to low doses of dihydrocodeine (up to 450 mgs daily). In some instances it may be preferable to substitute this level of opiate use with oral dihydrocodeine rather than with methadone, especially if the patient cannot tolerate methadone or is unwilling to take it.

These medications may also be considered for individuals who are travelling on holiday, as a temporary measure, because of their portability.

There are no formal studies to give empirical support to the effectiveness of dihydrocodeine in providing improved completion rates for detoxification, or other additional benefit.

---

c) Dihydrocodeine

3. Benzodiazepine

a) Benzodiazepine Reduction

Licensed for the management of benzodiazepine withdrawal.

Appropriate dosages of common benzodiazepines equivalent to 5mg of diazepam

Drug	Dose
Chlordiazepoxide	15 mg
Diazepam	5 mg
Loprazolam	500 microgram
Lorazepam	500 microgram
Oxazepam	15 mg
Temazepam	10 mg
Nitrazepam	5 mg

The following guidelines are suitable for a long-term benzodiazepine withdrawal regime in the community.[1]

i) Convert all benzodiazepines to diazepam, using the conversion chart above

Diazepam has several advantages over other benzodiazepines. It has a relatively long half-life and is available in different strength tablets. It can be given as a once a day dose which may need to be adjusted against withdrawal symptoms.

ii) How much to prescribe

■ As in any substitute prescribing, the doctor should aim for the lowest dose that will prevent withdrawal symptoms.

■ In cases of non-prescribed high-dose benzodiazepine abuse, the amount prescribed should be substantially less than the amount the patient claims to be taking.[2]

---

[1] Seivewright N., *Benzodiazepine Misuse*. Report for Department of Health Task Force to review services for drug misusers, 1995.
[2] Harrison M., Busto U., Naranjo C.A., Kaplan H.L., Sellers E.M., 'Diazepam tapering in detoxification for high-dose benzodiazepine abuse.' *Clinical Pharmacology and Therapeutics* 1984; **36**: 527–533.

■ Encourage the patient to divide the daily dose so as to avoid being intoxicated or drowsy during the day.

■ If very high dose prescribing is required the patient should be referred for specialist assessment.

■ The rate of withdrawal is often determined by an individual's capacity to tolerate symptoms. A benzodiazepine can be withdrawn in proportions of about one-eighth (range one-tenth to one-quarter) of daily dose every fortnight. In therapeutic dose dependence, the rate can be reduced by 2 to 2.5mg and if withdrawal symptoms occur then the dose can be maintained until symptoms improve. If the patient is not coping and is experiencing severe withdrawal symptoms, it may be necessary to increase the dose to alleviate the symptoms.

■ In cases where supra-therapeutic or high dose dependence occurs the practitioner needs to exert caution in their assessment and prescribing. If the patient is stable and free of withdrawal symptoms, at for example 50mg a day, the dose should be gradually reduced by half over 6 weeks and then reviewed. This rate of reduction led to no convulsions even in a group who had a high incidence of these during previous benzodiazepine withdrawals.[3] Practitioners suggest regimens that reduce the dose by 5–10mg per month, with smaller reductions at lower doses.[4]

■ If insomnia remains a problem, consider prescribing a non-benzodiazepine hypnotic for 2 weeks maximum, e.g. Perphenazine 4mg nocte.

iii) Adjunctive therapies

While reducing the dose, counselling, support groups and relaxation techniques can be helpful.

iv) Monitoring

It is important to note that because of long-term effects, all patients on a benzodiazepine prescription must be regularly reviewed, on at least a three-monthly basis.

If the patient on the benzodiazepine withdrawal regimen is also receiving a long-term prescription of methadone for concomitant opiate dependency, the methadone should be kept stable throughout the benzodiazepine reduction period. Concurrent detoxification in the community of both drugs is not recommended.

b) Dispensing

Where practicable, this should follow a schedule similar to that for other drugs of dependence.

---

[3] Scott R.T. 'The prevention of convulsions during benzodiazepine withdrawals.' *British Journal of General Practice* 1990; **40**: 261
[4] *Benzodiazepine Guidelines: Produced by Substance Misuse Project (SMP)*. Brent and Harrow Health Authority, 5 Jardine House, Harrovian Business Village. Bessborough Road, Harrow, Middx HA1 3EX.

4. Maintenance prescribing

a) Introduction

While some patients can achieve abstinence rapidly, others require the support of the prescribed drugs for longer than just a few months. Longer-term prescribing should be reviewed at regular intervals (at least 3-monthly) and should be part of a broader programme of social and psychological support. It should not be a treatment of first choice in a patient presenting for the first time, where other options have not initially been explored and tried.

Maintenance treatment with methadone

Opiate maintenance treatment is increasingly recognised to be an effective management strategy and oral methadone is the most commonly used drug. However, there is an increasing body of work reporting on the effectiveness of other agents, such as LAAM and buprenorphine, in the context of high quality, well supervised and well organised treatment services.

In most circumstances, but especially if the provision of a long-term prescription (e.g. for more than a few weeks) is proposed, local protocols and guidelines should be consulted and advice sought from a specialist (or specialised generalist).

If a decision to provide a long-term maintenance prescription is being considered, a number of factors which assist treatment effectiveness need to be incorporated:

i) Patients may need to be seen at least fortnightly initially and then, if stable, **at least monthly**.

ii) Random urine checks may be helpful, e.g. at least twice a year.

iii) Co-existing physical, emotional, social and legal problems, as well as drug and alcohol use, should be addressed as far as possible.

iv) A more thorough review every 3 months may be useful to consider what has been achieved and to set new goals.

Maintenance treatment with naltrexone

It is also possible to provide maintenance treatment with the opiate antagonist naltrexone, for those who have completed opiate withdrawal and require pharmacological assistance to maintain a drug-free state. Treatment compliance and supervision of medication appear to be critical in achieving good outcomes with naltrexone treatment.

b) Research evidence for methadone maintenance

The last Clinical Guidelines briefly mentioned methadone maintenance and considered it to be a specialised form of treatment best provided by a specialist drug misuse service, and then only for a small proportion of patients. The use of methadone maintenance now has a strong evidence base.[5, 6] Methadone maintenance is one of the most researched of the available treatment modalities and an overall assessment of its effectiveness can be made with more confidence than for other treatments.[7] If practitioners are properly trained, methadone maintenance can be effectively delivered in a wide range of settings, including primary care.

> *The 1993 ACMD Update report concluded that: "The benefit to be gained from oral methadone maintenance programmes both in terms of individual and public health and cost effectiveness has now been clearly demonstrated and we conclude that the development of structured programmes in the UK would represent a major improvement in this area of service delivery."*

A number of randomised controlled trials have been conducted, in which comprehensive methadone maintenance has been compared to a control condition over a substantial period of time, All of these trials found that on a number of measures (e.g. illicit opioid use, involvement in crime, mortality) methadone maintenance was vastly superior to control conditions.[8]

Taken together over two decades, the randomised studies of methadone maintenance demonstrate consistent, positive results over vastly different cultural contexts (US, Hong Kong, Sweden, Thailand). There have also been numerous observational studies demonstrating that the treatment delivered in many different settings confers substantial positive change. The one-year follow-up of the National Treatment Outcome Research Study, which is monitoring the progress of 1075 clients recruited into either residential or community treatment services over five years, also supports these findings.[9]

c) The effectiveness of methadone maintenance

Methadone maintenance (as delivered in structured programmes) is effective in reducing all of the following:

- Injecting behaviour
- Illicit opioid use
- Criminal activity
- Costs to society

---

[5] Farrell M., Ward I., Mattick R., *et al.* 'Methadone maintenance treatment in opiate dependence: a review.' *British Medical Journal* 1994; **309**: 997–1001.

[6] Ward J., Mattick R., Hall W., *Maintenance treatment and other opioid replacement therapies.* Harwood Academic Press, 1997.

[7] Marsch L.A., 'The efficacy of methadone maintenance interventions in reducing illicit opiate use, HIV risk behaviour and criminality: a meta-analysis.' *Addiction* 1998; **93**: 515–532.

[8] Ward J., Mattick R. and Hall W., *Maintenance treatment and other opioid replacement therapies.* Harwood Academic Press, 1997.

[9] Gossop M., Stewart D., Marsden J., *NTORS At One Year, The National Treatment Outcome Research Study: Changes in Substance Use, Health and Criminal Behaviours One Year after Intake.* London: Department of Health, 1998.

d) Conclusion

The Task Force to Review Services for Drug Misusers (1996) concluded that:

"The international evidence suggests that outpatient methadone maintenance programmes which incorporate psychosocial interventions can enable clients to remain stable and are effective in reducing drug misuse, improving health and reducing criminal activity. These programmes therefore form a significant component of drug misuse services."

e) Dosing regime for methadone maintenance

After careful dose induction (see earlier section on dose induction) and dose stabilisation, there is a consistent finding of greater benefit from maintaining individuals on a daily dose between 60mg and 120mg. In some instances, due to a patient's high tolerance, higher doses may be required but this is exceptional, such as where plasma methadone levels reveal persistent sub-therapeutic dosing even when compliance has been supervised. The use of plasma methadone monitoring can assist in determining the adequacy of dosage, particularly where the clinician has ensured that there is good compliance through supervised consumption.

High doses can reduce heroin and other opiate consumption, but caution needs to be observed about high doses if there is associated alcohol or benzodiazepine dependence. If patients miss methadone doses, for whatever reason, they need to be reassessed for intoxication and withdrawal before methadone administration is recommended. It may be appropriate to reduce the dose if the patient has not had methadone for more than 3 days, as their tolerance may be reduced.

If a patient has abstained from methadone for 5 days or more, they will require a full assessment before methadone is recommended.

5. Alternative opiate agonist agents

a) Levo-alpha-acetylmethadol (LAAM)

Not currently licensed for the management of drug dependence.

LAAM, in an oral preparation, is a congener of methadone and is a longer-acting alternative which can be given once every 2 to 3 days. The long-term effectiveness of LAAM with respect to reducing illegal drug misuse, criminality, HIV status and risk behaviours, appears to be comparable to methadone.[10,11] LAAM has the advantage that it can be taken less frequently. There is no experience to date of use in the UK and further studies will be needed to clarify its utility in the UK context. LAAM does not yet (at the time of preparation of the Department of Health Guidelines) have a Medicines Control Agency licence.

---

[10] Rawson R.A., Hasson A.L., Huber A.M., McCann M.J., Ling W., 'A 3-year progress report on the implementation of LAAM in the United States.' *Addiction* 1998; **93**: 533–40.
[11] Glanz M., Klawansky S., McAullife W., Chalmers T., 'Methadone vs. L-alpha-acetylmethadol (LAAM) in the treatment of opiate addiction. A meta-analysis of the randomized, controlled trials.' *American Journal of Addiction* 1997; **6**: 339–349.

b) Buprenorphine

Licensed for the management of drug dependence.

While buprenorphine abuse has been well recognised in the UK, there is now good evidence from overseas that, in the context of a well-supervised and well-monitored programme, buprenorphine can be useful as an alternative maintenance agent for those with lower levels of opiate dependence. There are a number of studies to support this (particularly from the USA), but to date, it has not been investigated seriously as a maintenance agent in the UK.

6. Injectable prescribing for maintenance purposes

a) General issues

No injectable preparations are licensed for use in the management of drug dependence.

This is a controversial area where further research is required to guide rational clinical practice. However, despite such lack of evidence, there is a view that a small number of long-term injectors can benefit from such prescribing.[12, 13] The idea that prescribing injectables is one point on a continuum, which has being drug free at its opposite end, is attractive, but it is clear that many doctors experience great difficulty in moving patients along the desired treatment path.

There are currently no clear criteria to guide such decision making but repeated failure within existing treatment regimens is the most commonly quoted instance. Failure to engage previously in any form of treatment in the context of severe and long-standing problems can also give rise to consideration of use of injectable medication. When a clinician embarks on such prescribing it should be against a background of a long and persistent history of injecting drug use, and in all cases there should be clear goals that can be assessed at defined intervals.

Means should exist to supervise and monitor, in a clinical setting, the administration of the drug in the early stages of treatment, and at later stages where concern over clinical progress arises. Where pharmacy dispensing occurs, it should be daily to reduce the risk of diversion. Where evidence of diversion exists, daily supervised forms of medication should be re-established.

In the absence of demonstrated significant superior outcomes from this form of clinical practice, and in recognition of the greater inherent dangers and the cost burden of such prescribing, services should regularly audit and review outcomes against set performance standards.

Specialists prescribing injectable formulations should bear in mind that, once initiated, they are likely to become a long-term clinical commitment. Such a long-term high resource commitment needs to be taken into consideration when initiating such prescribing.

There is no recognised indication for prescribing injectable amphetamines, cocaine or benzodiazepines.

---

[12] Martin E., 'Prescribing injectable opiates. Substance Misuse Management in General Practice,' *Newsletter issue No 4*, 1997.
[13] Department of Health. *Task Force to review services for drug misusers: report of an Independent Review of Drug Treatment Services in England.* London: Department of Health, 1996. (Chairman: The Reverend Dr John Polkinghorne)

b) Injectable methadone

Injectable methadone has a very high currency in the illicit market, therefore all the clinical issues contributing to compliance and security apply particularly to this form of the drug.

These could include:

- daily dispensing in most situations;

- regular monitoring of the patient's condition;

- the use of plasma methadone levels.

Prescribing injectable methadone is a clinical decision to be made on the basis of the suitability of the individual patient.

The following issues relating to the patient should be taken into account:

- is this an appropriate manner of patient engagement?

- if there is evidence of poly-substance misuse, including alcohol dependency, the risks of overdose need serious consideration;

- determination and persistence of patient to continue injecting;

- severe opiate dependence;

- reasonable venous access;

- absence of deep vein thrombosis and related pathologies;

- evidence of reasonable knowledge of the principles of safe injecting.

Additionally, the following issues, relating to the prescriber, should be considered:

- The level of training defining competence to prescribe injectable methadone.

- Are there reasonable, clearly defined and measurable patient goals within a broader psychosocial framework?

- The appropriate Home Office licence may be required to prescribe injectable methadone.

Conclusions

- There is a very limited clinical place for prescribing injectable methadone.

- There are no simple criteria for prescribing injectables, but rather a complex clinical decision based on the suitability of each individual patient.

- Prescribing injectables has costs (prolonging dependence, collusion with the drug culture, problems of misuse and diversion) and so the benefits (health gain, reduced criminality, engaging more entrenched drug misusers) must be clear.

c) Diamorphine (heroin)

A short-acting opiate agonist, mainly used intravenously, but can also be taken in oral form and inhaled. It is used as part of a maintenance regime in a minority of patients. A Home Office licence is required for such prescribing, which is the preserve of specialists. Diamorphine should only be prescribed in situations of rigorous monitoring and where use in the initial stages can be supervised. With the availability of injectable methadone, there is very little clinical indication for prescribed diamorphine. All the caveats and criteria discussed with regard to injectable methadone apply to diamorphine.

7. Naltrexone

Naltrexone can be taken orally and blocks the effects of opiates for up to 72 hours. Patients need to be warned that an attempt to overcome the block could result in acute opioid intoxication.

Induction: Some clinicians use a naloxone challenge test to confirm opiate drug-free status in the absence of naloxone-induced opiate withdrawal before starting the naltrexone regimen. This should be done 10 days after the last reported opiate consumed. If done over a shorter time interval, there is a greater risk of precipitating withdrawal symptoms. A challenge of 0.4–1.2mg intravenous naloxone should be given and, if negative, then a test dose of 12.5 or 25mg of naltrexone can be given.

Dose: 25mg initially then 50mg daily; the total weekly dose may be divided and given on 3 days of the week for improved compliance (e.g. 100mg on Monday, Wednesday, and 150mg on Friday), but many patients prefer daily dosing.

Training and support to enhance compliance with medication can include family and couple work where appropriate. This is to enhance strategies for supervision of medication consumption.

8. Summary

Prescribing for dependence or withdrawal

Pharmacological group	Drug	Licence status for the treatment of drug dependency
Opiates		
	Methadone mixture or oral methadone in a liquid form (such as methadone mixture 1mg/ml)	LICENSED
	Lofexidine	LICENSED
	Naltrexone	LICENSED FOR RELAPSE PREVENTION
	Buprenorphine	LICENSED
	Dihydrocodeine, Codeine	NOT LICENSED
	LAAM	NOT LICENSED
	Diamorphine (heroin)	NOT LICENSED
Benzodiazepines		
	Diazepam	LICENSED FOR BENZODIAZEPINE WITHDRAWAL
	Chlordiazepoxide	LICENSED FOR ALCOHOL WITHDRAWAL
Stimulants		
Amphetamines	Dexamphetamine	NOT LICENSED
Cocaine	Antidepressants (e.g. fluoxetine)	LICENSED FOR DEPRESSION

CHAPTER 7
PREVENTING RELAPSE

Key chapter recommendations

> The clinician has a responsibility to ensure that the patient receives the correct dose and that appropriate efforts are taken to ensure that the drug is used appropriately and not diverted onto the illegal market.

> As well as opiate maintenance and detoxification prescribing, clinicians need to be aware of the potential benefits of prescribing opiate antagonists, such as naltrexone, for the prevention of relapse in those who have achieved abstinence. Strategies for the induction and maintenance of naltrexone should be a treatment option shared between specialised and primary care services.

> Clinicians need to understand the crucial role of broader psychosocial interventions in achieving and maintaining abstinence. Such an approach will usually involve multidisciplinary team care.

> The management of drug misuse and dependence presents a considerable clinical challenge to all practitioners. However, well delivered treatment with good outcomes enhances the clinician's competence and confidence in tackling these complex problems to the benefit of the individual patient and to society.

> As with all interventions, pragmatic clinicians need to take a realistic view of the range of outcomes possible with this type of problem.

1.   Introduction

Withdrawal and detoxification regimens have a high failure rate unless linked to long-term rehabilitation. Nevertheless, complying with the overall treatment package is the key to treatment success and monitoring progress along these lines is critical. Failure to identify and address non-compliance at an early stage can result in loss of therapeutic endeavour and the will to change on behalf of the patient. Non-compliance with prescribed medication can actually aggravate a person's drug problem.[1]

---

[1] Department of Health. *The Task Force to review services for drug misusers: report of an Independent Survey of Drug Treatment Services In England.* London: Department of Health, 1996. (Chairman: The Reverend Dr John Polkinghorne)

2. Consequences of non-compliance

■ The patient may take an excess of the drug and risk overdose.

■ The drug may get into the wrong hands, risking the safety and well-being of others.

■ The patient may sell the drug to purchase other illicit drugs, thereby perpetuating controlled drug misuse and contributing to the illicit market.[2]

■ Diversion of methadone into the illicit market may contribute significantly to risks of death from overdose. Methadone, dihydrocodeine and a variety of benzodiazepines, are readily available on the illicit market in many parts of the United Kingdom.

3. Improving compliance

a) Assessment during treatment

Arrange to see the patient weekly in the first few weeks. Though change will occur slowly, a weekly consultation gives a valuable opportunity to build up a relationship of trust and understanding. Once a patient is stable, fortnightly or monthly appointments may be sufficient. A full review should be undertaken every three months.

If prescribing a substitute drug, is the dose sufficient?

■ Look for signs of withdrawal or toxicity. Encourage feedback from the community pharmacist and other professionals who may be seeing the patient more frequently.

Is the patient continuing to misuse illegal drugs?

■ If the patient is continuing to inject drugs, despite the obvious health risks, ensure that he/she is obtaining sterile needles and syringes. It may be that the patient continues illegal drug misuse because doses of the substitute drug are insufficient. Continued injecting use can be confirmed by physical examination of injecting sites.

Is the substitute drug dose inadequate?

■ Consider increasing the dose by small increments on a daily or weekly basis until the signs of withdrawal have disappeared and misuse of illegal drugs reduces or ceases.

■ Do not continue to increase the dose if there are signs of intoxication.

■ Randomised and/or supervised collection of urine specimens every few months may be helpful.

---

[2] Fountain J., Griffiths P., Farrell M., Gossop M., Strang J., 'Diversion tactics: how a sample of drug misusers in treatment obtained surplus drugs to sell on the illicit market.' *The International Journal of Drug Policy* 1997; **9**: 159–167.

- Keep a careful note of the use of any unauthorised drugs (type, quantity and route) and ask about any legal, medical or social changes.

- Review treatment goals regularly, on **at least a three-monthly basis**.

b) Supervised consumption

Supervised consumption with an appropriate professional provides the best guarantee that the drug is being taken as directed.

- In most cases, all new patients being prescribed methadone should be required to take their daily dose under the direct supervision of a professional for a period of time which may, depending on the individual patient, be at least 3 months, subject to compliance.

- Similarly, when the patient restarts methadone after a break, or receives a significant increase in the methadone dose, daily dispensing, ideally with supervised consumption, should be re-instated for a period of time agreed in local guidelines and protocols.

- These arrangements should only be relaxed, so as to allow take-home doses, if the doctor can be satisfied that compliance will be maintained. The relaxation of supervision can be seen as an important component of rehabilitation and re-establishing acceptable responsible behaviour.

- Arrangements for daily dispensing through instalment prescribing, and where appropriate, supervised consumption of other drugs, should also be made.

Take-home doses should not be prescribed where:

- the patient shows a continued and unstable, or unauthorised, pattern of drug misuse, including a significant increase in alcohol intake, the use of illicit drugs, benzodiazepines or other tranquillizers;

- the patient has a significant unstable psychiatric illness;

- there is continuing concern that the prescribed drug is being diverted or used inappropriately.

Other methods for improving compliance:

i)   **Urine testing.** Random urinalysis may encourage compliance.

ii)   **Daily pick-up.** Requiring the patient to collect his or her dose each day may increase compliance by restricting the dose dispensed, but still provides no guarantee that the drug will be taken as directed.

iii) **Instalment prescribing.** Wherever possible, substitute drugs used in treatment should be written on prescription forms that allow for daily or instalment dispensing.

c) Improving patient attendance

Drug misusers respond best when they are treated like any other patients and are able to keep appointments on time, if it is part of a clear treatment contract. It may be easier for them to comply where late appointments or a drop-in system are available.

d) Naltrexone

The use of the pure opiate antagonist, naltrexone, to assist relapse prevention has been explored for the last three decades.[3, 4] The prophylactic use of such a drug, which blocks all opiate effects, would therefore precipitate uncomfortable or severe opiate withdrawal symptoms if taken by an individual dependent on opiates. Use of heroin or other opiates by an individual maintained on naltrexone, is not associated with any positive or euphoric effect, because of the naltrexone opiate receptor blockade.

Naltrexone-assisted relapse prevention should only be initiated by specialists and specialised generalists experienced in this technique. Where it is set up, shared care arrangements should be clearly delineated, between the specialist and the patient's general practitioner. Ideally, community drug services should provide a naltrexone challenge and naltrexone induction service that can be continued in an appropriate community setting.

Further work is needed to explore the use of naltrexone in a community setting.

4. Non-pharmacological approaches to relapse prevention

A number of behavioural techniques have been developed to prevent relapse. Typically, these involve the identification of high-risk situations, where there is an increased likelihood of drug taking behaviour. Rehabilitation and therapeutic communities are treatments aimed at developing specific changes in lifestyle to remain drug free in an environment where drugs are easily available. Self-help groups, such as Narcotics Anonymous (NA), aim to help drug-dependent or drug taking individuals become abstinent. An important component of NA programmes is the adoption of limited objectives. The individual is advised to promise him/herself not to use drugs for just one day, something that many have done willingly or unwillingly in the past and therefore know to be possible. Having abstained for one day, the individual renews this short achievable contract with themself. If a day is too long, then the time can be shortened to just 10 minutes at a time. This strategy focuses the person's mind on the immediate problem of not taking drugs and undermines practised excuses and the rationalisation for drug taking.

[3] Gonzalez J.P., Brogden R.N., 'Naltrexone. A review of its pharmacodynamic and pharmacokinetic properties and therapeutic efficacy in the management of opioid dependence.' *Drugs* 1988; **35**: 192-213.

[4] Shufman E.N., Porat S., Witztum E., Gandacu D., Bar-Hamburger R., Ginath Y., 'The efficacy of naltrexone in preventing reabuse of heroin after detoxification.' *Biological Psychiatry* 1994; **35**: 935-945.

5. Broader approaches to psychosocial support and treatment

While much of these Guidelines has focused on aspects of the medical management of drug dependence, it is important that such management be seen within a broader context of possible options for intervention and support. As well as specialist drug services, there is also a range of more generic help available such as that for victims of trauma, while counselling and mental health services should also be considered.

Many people with serious drug and alcohol problems will have a complex range of other problems that will require support, usually in the context of shared care and individual counselling. However, for some, more intensive support will be required and the option of community care assessment should be considered, in order to seek appropriate support for day care or residential care.

For some, a crisis may occur that requires immediate intervention, which may necessitate admission. Notwithstanding limited resources, referral to hospital or residential service may assist in addressing problems that have become unmanageable in a community setting.

Community Care Assessment can be accessed through local Social Service Departments. Such services have some funding to purchase residential or day programmes for individuals, after appropriate assessment.

There are currently 100 residential services listed for England and Wales, examples being:

- Twelve Step – based on Narcotics Anonymous.

- Concept House – based on a hierarchical model derived from the early rehabilitation movement in the United States.

- A range of Christian, Buddhist and other religious communities, which provide services with a focus on community living, counselling and general development, as part of a way of moving away from a drug-using lifestyle.

There are also an increasing number of day programmes for:

– drug misusing offenders

– vocational training

– post-residential rehabilitation programmes.

There is an evolving range of care being developed that focuses on broader aspects of drug users' lifestyles. These can be invaluable for the patient if a meaningful engagement with the service can be achieved.

ANNEX 1
SHARED WORKING WITH OTHER PROFESSIONALS

1. Multiprofessional

The emphasis in these Guidelines is on the rich potential for multidisciplinary and shared working. There are a range of professionals who come into contact with drug users as part of their daily work and who can provide valuable support and advice to the Primary Care Team. There is a considerable resource of people who are ready and willing to work jointly around some of these complex problems. Within a range of shared care models, community drug and alcohol team workers can provide: consultation-liaison, advice, brief assessment, joint clinics, satellite clinics and a range of other services as part of a primary care support service. Others will provide training for practice managers, receptionists and other primary health care team members on approaches to managing drug users in a general practice setting.

Nurses and drug workers provide most of the community-based drug services and they are major contributors to shared care. Pharmacists and social workers are other key professionals with intensive contact with drug users.

An effective community-based service depends on the close working relationships of these professionals.

2. Role of the nurse

Nurses work in many different settings with drug misusers, and have many different approaches to care, often as members of multidisciplinary teams with direct contact with medical practitioners. Their skills and techniques range from assessment of drug misusers, counselling, carrying out other treatment procedures, to health education and teaching. Their clinical and treatment role in drug misuse services is as varied as it is essential.

The role of the nurse has expanded enormously over the last few years. This expansion is laid out in recent White Papers and further developed through the formation of Primary Care Groups and their equivalents. For nurses working with drug and alcohol users, a series of guidance documents have been published by the Association of Nurses in Substance Abuse (ANSA).

In 1997, ANSA published, with the endorsement of the Department of Health's Chief Nursing Officer, guidance documents for specialist nurses working with drug and alcohol users.[1]

3. Role of the drugs worker

In the drug misuse field, workers from a variety of professional backgrounds, including teaching, nursing, social work and the criminal justice system, are often referred to as drugs counsellors or drugs workers. Many drugs workers are found in voluntary agencies working with drug misusers, and indeed form the core personnel of these services. Their professional function can be considered as the major part of the full range of psychosocial services required for comprehensive treatment.

Drugs workers often provide support, advice and basic counselling for drug misusers, may act as the patient/client's key worker, and carry a caseload similar to a social worker. They may be involved in outreach and befriending work, needle exchange schemes, street services, day services and various residential services.

Almost all drugs workers provide basic counselling but some are trained in specific counselling techniques including individual, family therapies and working with young people. Counselling drug misusers is a core function in treatment and rehabilitation services, and professional competence and clinical effectiveness is closely related to training, competent supervision and formal accreditation. Drugs workers practise in a 'social work model' and can address family and personal relationships, child-care, housing, income support and criminal justice issues.

4. Role of the clinical psychologist

Clinical psychology can play a major role in the treatment of drug misuse. Psychological theory provides models of explanation of dependent behaviour, which complements neurobiological and social theories. Psychological techniques, which directly address behaviours, cognition and decision-making, have become a central part of good clinical practice in the treatment of drug misuse and are important adjuncts to pharmacotherapy. For example, motivational interviewing strategies may be important in the initial assessment to engage drug misusers in services. For individuals planning detoxification/withdrawal, relapse prevention strategies often need to be an integrated part of treatment. Individuals with co-existing mental health and drug misuse problems can also benefit from specific psychological therapies e.g. cognitive behavioural.

---

[1] *Working Within Primary Health Care Teams* (1997) ANSA; *Working With Children & Young People* (1997) ANSA; *Working With Alcohol and Drug Users* (1997) ANSA.
Publications can be obtained from: Pinpoint Communications Ltd
12 Skene Road, Kingston upon Thames, Surrey KT2 5AP,
Tel: 0181 547 1810, Fax: 0181 974 5773

5. Role of the community and hospital pharmacists

Community pharmacist

Community pharmacists provide a significant point of contact as part of primary health care services and have regular (often daily) contact with the patient. Hence their role in the care of drug misusers is crucial, and communication in both directions between pharmacists and other health care professionals should be encouraged.

Specifically, community pharmacists can offer the following services for drug misusers: dispensing controlled drugs prescriptions; monitoring prescriptions for drug interactions and adverse drug reactions; supplying clean injecting equipment, whether by sale or through needle exchange; referring clients to drug treatment agencies; providing verbal and written information and advice. Community pharmacists are also ideally placed to monitor prescriptions for potential over-use of medicines using patient medication records; they can additionally evaluate the legal validity of prescriptions and screen prescriptions for errors. The community pharmacist can play an important role in identifying inappropriate prescribing of controlled drugs and monitoring the misuse potential of 'over the counter' medicines.

Community pharmacists are not obliged to supervise the self-administration of controlled drugs by the patient in the pharmacy, although many are willing to do so. It is recommended that pharmacists who are willing to provide this service are adequately trained and have suitable guidance relating to when and if to withhold a dose of the drug. This could cover, for example, cases where patients have missed treatment for a number of days consecutively or when a patient attends the pharmacy intoxicated.

Hospital pharmacist

Hospital pharmacists have an important role in advising general hospital clinicians when a patient, maintained on substitute medication, is admitted whether to accident and emergency or as a planned medical or surgical admission.

The hospital pharmacist can:

i)   Advise clinicians of possible interactions with methadone and other medications.

ii)   Give advice as to how a patient's substitute medication regime can be continued appropriately, either on admission or in preparation for discharge.

iii) Advise on the practicalities of issuing instruction to nursing staff when controlled drugs are being prescribed.

iv)   For outpatient populations, the hospital pharmacist has a role in communicating and liaising with hospital, community and primary care professionals.

The code of ethics of the Royal Pharmaceutical Society of Great Britain (RPSGB) directs pharmacists to maintain client/patient confidentiality. However, clients should be made aware that, in certain circumstances, the pharmacist may communicate information about compliance to the prescriber. Clear guidance is needed about what may be communicated to the prescriber without the patient's consent.

Recommended reading: *Report of the Working Party on Pharmaceutical Services for Drug Misusers.* London: Royal Pharmaceutical Society of Great Britain, 1998.

6. Role of the social worker

Social workers in local authority Social Service Departments (SSDs) bring general social work skills into many community and residential settings where there are drug misusers. They are particularly involved when there are child and family care issues which place children in vulnerable circumstances.

In recent years, some SSDs have identified a key social work officer to co-ordinate social work responses and resources for drug misusers, and some authorities have encouraged the development of specialist social workers attached to specialist multidisciplinary drug misuse teams.

Since the introduction of the National Health Service and Community Care Act 1990, social work staff have played a central role in allocating the provision of longer-term residential rehabilitation for drug misusers through their role in providing community care assessments.

Community care assessment can also explore possible options for support in a non-residential setting. Referral for community care assessment can be a source of additional support for individuals who have complex needs.

ANNEX 2
TRAINING FOR CLINICIANS WORKING WITH DRUG MISUSERS

Training for the generalist

This annex focuses on the training needs of 'generalists'. These are GPs who provide assessment, detoxification and prescribing services, wherever possible within the context of a shared care agreement with a specialised generalist or generalist provider.

1.   Introduction

Training programmes should address the different levels of involvement of primary health care teams and be sufficiently flexible to meet the demands of local conditions.

> **The health authority or health board is responsible for ensuring the availability of support for primary health care teams. Training is a crucial element in that support.**

The following principles should underpin the development of all training:

- ■   Training should be undertaken in a planned way.

- ■   Wherever possible, training should result in a formal recognition of competence.

- ■   Training should be delivered by tutors with specialist skills and knowledge appropriate to the needs of primary health care teams. In most cases this will be led by a tutor from the same professional background.

2.   Training for the wider Primary Health Care Team (PHCT)

Training must address not only the needs of GPs but also those of front-line reception staff, managers and other clinical members of the primary health care team.

3. A training curriculum for primary care

At the end of this annex is a suggested set of topics to be covered, which will deliver basic competency in treating drug misusers in primary care within a shared care agreement. This attempts to highlight the issues which the PHCT will need to be aware of as a minimum, notwithstanding different training requirements for different members of the primary health care team.

a) Delivery of training

Training should be delivered locally, with the involvement of local specialist providers based, where appropriate, on any national training guidelines or material and the core topics listed below, but taking into account the needs of the PHCT and local circumstances. There is no optimum length for a training course but experience suggests that an appropriate package might take *in total* around three days. The length of time over which training takes place will vary but, if the training is spread over a longer period than about six months, some of the benefits may be lost.

b) Accreditation

Some form of accreditation and continuous audit of local training will need to be in place. This should be developed within the local context and health authorities should consider how best to develop accreditation locally. Local accreditation should create a structure within which individual practitioners and PHCTs can enter into locally developed shared care schemes and a means of monitoring the quality of shared care. Schemes will assess the appropriateness of training courses, the suitability of methods of delivery and the competence of trainers. Accreditation of training should be combined with monitoring of subsequent practice, thereby establishing continuous evaluation of training schemes. Local accreditation and monitoring should be overseen by a senior medical figure, e.g. the Director of Public Health.

4. Proposed curriculum for shared care training

Background issues

The prevalence and nature of the drug problem nationally and locally.

Drugs and the law, legislation, national policy, national guidance.

Who uses drugs and why?

Recreational and problem drug use.

The nature of dependence.

The role of shared care and primary care in treating drug misusers

Shared care: what is it?

Who should be managed in general practice?

Local treatment arrangements.

The role of specialist services.

Integrating drug misusers and the practice population.

Impact on other practice activity.

The role of non-medical staff.

Managing and avoiding aggressive behaviour.

Providing information to the Regional Drug Misuse Database.

Treatment issues

Treating different drug misusers:
- opiate misusers
- amphetamines misusers
- cocaine misusers
- benzodiazepine misusers
- misusers of other drugs, e.g, volatile substances
- alcohol and drug misusers

General prescribing issues

The role of urine testing

Assessment

Detoxification

Injecting behaviour and advice

Other techniques:
- the role of counselling
- motivational interviewing

Complex cases and multiple dependencies:
- dual diagnosis
- HIV/hepatitis B & C
- young people
- drug misuse and pregnancy

Prescribing in primary care

Using the Clinical Guidelines

The role and purpose of substitute prescribing

Principles and protocols for substitute prescribing

Prescribing methadone

- – in what circumstances?
- – what formulation?
- – how much to prescribe?
- – reduction and maintenance
- – managing the stable methadone user
- – when to refer to a specialist service

Prescribing other substitute drugs

Prescribing and the law – who can prescribe what?

Preventing 'leakage'

The role of the pharmacist

The role of other professions and agencies

The range of other professions and services locally

Specialist services

Community Drugs Teams

Social Services

Pharmacists

Needle exchanges

Probation

Police

Education

Wider health issues

General health issues for drug misusers

Harm reduction and primary prevention

Blood-borne viruses:

– HIV/AIDS

– hepatitis B, including vaccinations

– hepatitis C

Other problems with injecting

ANNEX 3
HEALTH AND SAFETY/MANAGING CHALLENGING BEHAVIOUR

1.   Avoiding the violent or dangerous situation

In settings where drug misusing patients are seen and treated, it is important that staff have a clear policy of action to follow if they are confronted by disruptive or threatening behaviour. However, well-organised and properly supported GP surgeries are rarely troubled by any significant disruption.

Procedures and processes should be in place to cover the worst scenarios, especially when hazards exist in combination, such as giving bad news to someone with a history of violence, or consulting alone in a late evening or Saturday surgery.

Procedures should address and clarify the following points:

- What is the attitude to drug misusers attending appointments accompanied by groups of friends?

- What action should be taken in the event of:
  – patients shouting at receptionists, nurses or other patients?
  – patients threatening receptionists, nurses or other patients?
  – patients being violent?

- In which situations should the police be called.

2.   GP surgery/A&E

i)   If a member of staff is working alone then reception staff should check if an appointment overruns. Equally, staff should notify reception of any delays that can be anticipated.

ii)   Avoid seeing patient alone who has been aggressive or threatening to staff or who is judged by reception staff to be clearly upset or angry whilst waiting. If unavoidable, inform reception staff and ask them to make periodic 'checks'.

iii)   Health care workers should keep potential 'weapons', such as sharps, out of reach and sight of a potentially violent patient.

iv)   Always keep a clear exit route by positioning yourself nearest to the door.

v)   If a patient is threatening or disruptive in the waiting room, it is useful to have a small room away from public view in which the patient can be seen by staff.

vi)   Safety equipment, such as mobile phones and assistance alarms, whilst not a panacea, should be available. Staff should be trained in how to respond to an alarm call.

vii) Predictably difficult consultations should be carried out in open areas, or with someone else present.

3. Home visits

i)   If the nurse or doctor is unsure of their safety on entering, they should consider opening up their mobile phone to the surgery and having the first few minutes of the consultation monitored.

ii)   Be alert when visiting someone at home for the first time.

iii) On home visits, be prepared not to enter premises or to leave if confronted with potential or actual violence. Alternative arrangements for attending to the patient can be made, which may involve a revisit with the police.

iv)   Request that dogs are removed to another room.

v)   GPs, Out of Hours Co-operatives and commercial deputising services should have clear guidelines as to the situation where they are willing to offer substitute controlled drugs for the treatment of addiction. These should follow those set out under the accident and emergency guidelines.

4. Information to patients

i)   Be consistent. Once the treatment setting has an agreed policy it is important to explain to all patients what the policy is and to be consistent in its application. For example, where receptionists and other administrative staff are expected to be firm in their application of the policy, it is important that they are supported by more senior staff.

ii)   It is important for the practitioner to know that giving in to demands is often not helpful, and indeed can be undermining for a patient who is actually expecting the security of a firm decision. Thus it is most important if 'no' is the decision to confidently follow it through. Later, the drug misuser may return to the doctor and positively acknowledge the firmness.

iii) If the behaviour is clearly unmanageable within available resources, it potentially becomes a criminal matter. This should be made quite clear to the patient and if the patient fails to co-operate, the police should be called to remove the patient. Where theft or clearly witnessed unacceptable behaviour or injury has taken place, it may be more valuable to press criminal charges than to appear to avoid the inconvenience of legal confrontation.

iv)   The message of a firm course of action soon gets communicated to other patients, making recurrence of the unacceptable behaviour much less likely.

5. Needlestick injuries

Needlestick injury is a rare occupational hazard for those working with drug misusers. Blood-borne viral infection is the main area of risk: HIV, hepatitis B and hepatitis C. It has been broadly estimated that a penetrating needlestick injury gives a 1 in 3 chance of acquiring hepatitis B, a 1 in 30 chance of acquiring hepatitis C and a 1 in 300 chance of acquiring HIV.

Immediate action should be taken following the needlestick or similar injury:

- Encourage bleeding at the site of the injury.
- Wash the injury thoroughly with warm running water and soap.
- Cover the injury site with plaster.
- Take a baseline blood sample for storage.
- Assess the risk of HIV or hepatitis transmission.
- Consider the need for prophylaxis against hepatitis B or HIV.

a) Hepatitis B

Staff members should be adequately protected in advance through immunisation. If an individual, who is not known to be immune, suffers a needlestick injury and the source of possibly infectious blood is positive or of unknown status, give hepatitis B immunoglobulin. If the patient is not immune, commence a hepatitis B vaccination programme.

b) Hepatitis C

Currently (1999), there is no prophylaxis available.

c) HIV

Any action should be guided by current accepted practice.

ANNEX 4
MODELS OF CHANGE

1. A natural history and drug career perspective

Clinical management must be considered in the context of the natural history of drug misuse. Awareness of the different stages drug misusers pass through can help the clinician make the right responses. For example, the needs of a young person under 20 years, newly involved in drug misuse, are very different when compared with an individual who has been injecting for over 20 years.

The natural history of most regular drug users is like that of the general population, with general reductions in consumption and increased cessation rates with age. There are many social pressures dissuading adults from ongoing drug use and the social consequences of ongoing heavy drug use result in significant marginalisation of those who persist in use. Thus many older drug misusers are well motivated to accept treatment. Most young people who take drugs stop as part of growing up. However, rates of cessation among dependent opiate users are significantly lower, but long-term studies are reported mainly from treatment populations.

2. The stages of change model applied to drug misuse

The stages of change model described by Prochaska and DiClemente, linked to the technique of motivational interviewing, has important practical applications for assessment and treatment.[1] Motivation is considered to be a pre-condition for effective treatment and this model assists the clinician to encourage motivation in a more effective way.[2,3]

The model recognises that established drug misusers often only actively engage in change, or treatment for change, when they have passed through various key stages.

- ■ **Pre-contemplation**: A stage where drug misusers are not aware that they have a problem, and therefore do not seriously think about change. It is others who recognise that there are problems and that change is required.

- ■ **Contemplation**: A stage where the individual begins to weigh up the pros and cons of their drug misuse; they feel somewhat ambivalent about their behaviour. The person considers that there might be a problem and that change might be necessary.

---

[1] Prochaska J.O., Diclemente C.C., 'Towards a Comprehensive Model of Change' in Miller W.R., Heather N., (eds) *Treating Addictive Behaviours, Processes of Change*. New York: Plenum Press, 1986: 3–27
[2] Miller W.R., 'Why do people change addictive behaviour? The 1996 H. David Archibald Lecture.' *Addiction* 1998; **93**: 163–172.
[3] Marlatt G.A., Gordon J.R., *Relapse prevention: maintenance strategies in the treatment of addictive behaviors.* New York: Guildford Press, 1985.

■ **Decision**: A hypothetical stage where the balance of change is influenced and a point is reached where a decision is made to do something, or possibly nothing, about their attendant behaviour.

■ **Action**: The process or stage of doing something. The person chooses a strategy for change and pursues it, taking steps to put their decision into effect. This is traditionally where 'motivation' for treatment would begin.

■ **Maintenance**: During this stage the task is to maintain the gains that have been made in order to avoid a return to undesired previous behaviours. Failure to consolidate progress may result in a relapse.

■ **Relapse**: At a point of relapse, the individual would return to previous patterns of behaviour at either a pre-contemplative, or contemplative stage. However, relapse in itself would not be considered a treatment failure but a positive learning experience, potentially increasing the successful outcome next time round.

i)   Pre-contemplation may last for years but practitioners and services can encourage the move to the contemplation stage, e.g. using specific forms of motivational interviewing and providing basic harm reduction advice. Contemplators also need encouragement to make a decision and enter the action phase of treatment e.g. detoxification, regular clinic attendance etc. Maintaining the positive effect of treatment involves structured and active follow-up to build on changes already made. This may take months or years.

ii) The model highlights that at each stage of treatment and change, misusers may relapse and return to previous phases. In the NTORS study the majority of drug misusers had already been in treatment in the two years before inclusion into the cohort and many had previous relapses.[4]

iii) The value of this model is that it assists in clarifying which stage the individual drug misuser is at and this informs the clinical response. It follows that clinical interventions must be tailored for particular stages and needs in a drug misuser's life. For example, there is no strong clinical indication to offer a substitute opioid drug or a package of detoxification to a drug misuser at the stage of pre-contemplation. However, there is a clinical responsibility to encourage the client to begin to contemplate his problem.

3. Using the Care Pathway Approach

Managing the complex needs of the drug misuser may require careful co-ordination of different professionals and levels of specialist drug agency input.

A structured Care Pathway Approach can be valuable to this co-ordination. This approach formally identifies a common series of treatment milestones (often related to the model of change discussed above), e.g. assessment, prescribing, review, rehabilitation, etc, which are operationally related to specific interventions by specific trained personnel in different agencies. The value of this approach is that it assists co-ordination and evaluation in what may be a complex clinical process.

---

[4] *The National Treatment Outcomes Research Study, summary of the project, the clients, and preliminary findings.* London: Department of Health, 1996.

ANNEX 5
PREGNANCY AND NEONATAL CARE

A district policy involving obstetricians, paediatricians, midwives, drug services, general practice and social service representatives can be very useful in establishing local guidelines for management of drug-using mothers.

1. Introduction

The number of women misusing drugs has increased considerably in the past 30 years, and many are in their child-bearing years.

Though pregnancy may act as a catalyst for change, drug misusers may not use general health services until late into pregnancy[1] and this increases the health risks for both the mother and child.[2]

Attracting and maintaining these women in treatment services is vital[3] as follow-up studies also suggest that the long-term outcome in women who enter methadone treatment programmes during pregnancy is better in terms of their pregnancy, childbirth and infant development, irrespective of continuing illicit drug misuse.[4,5] Women attending treatment services usually have better antenatal care and better general health than drug-using women not in treatment, even if they are still using illicit drugs.[6]

Engagement of the partner is an important aspect of enabling the pregnant women to achieve progress at the earliest possible stage.

2. Management by a multidisciplinary team

Different approaches have been tried to deliver care to pregnant drug misusers, such as specialist midwives, or drug dependence staff attached to the antenatal clinic.[7,8] Each method should try to involve the primary health care team, particularly if prescribing substitute medication.

---

[1] Klee H., Lewis S., Jackson M., *Illicit drug use in pregnancy and early motherhood: an analysis of the impediments to effective service delivery*. A Report prepared for the Department of Health, 1995.

[2] Faugier J., Hayes C., and Butterworth C.A., *Drug using prostitutes, their health care needs, and their clients*. Manchester: University of Manchester, 1992.

[3] Hepburn M., 'Drug misuse in pregnancy.' *British Journal of Hospital Medicine* 1993; **49**: 51–55.

[4] Finnegan L.P., 'Treatment issues for opioid-dependent women during the perinatal period.' *Journal of Psychoactive Drugs* 1991; **23**: 191–201.

[5] Fraser A., Cavanagh S., 'Pregnancy and drug addiction – long-term consequences.' *Journal of the Royal Society of Medicine* 1991; **84**: 530–532.

[6] Batey R.G., Weissel K., 'A 40 month follow-up of pregnant drug-using women treated at Westmead Hospital.' *Drug and Alcohol Review* 1993; **12**: 265–270.

[7] Dawe S., Gerada C., Strang J., Establishment of a liaison service for pregnant opiate-dependent women. *British Journal of Addiction* 1992; **87**: 867–871.

[8] London M., Caldwell R., 'Services for pregnant drug users.' *Psychol Bulletin* 1990; **14**: 12–15.

Annex 5 Pregnancy and Neonatal Care

The type of service in each area will depend on local circumstances, the number of pregnant drug misusers presenting for care, expertise of the obstetric and primary care services, and availability of specialist or shared-care support.

Obstetric departments should develop good links with local drug specialists and GPs and the local social services. Local statutory authorities should have a written policy about drug-misusing parents, and all professionals involved should be aware of the policy.

3. Management of antenatal care

The key aims of management are to attract the women into health care treatment services, provide antenatal care and stabilise or reduce drug use to the lowest possible dose.

Good co-ordination between relevant parties is important and child protection issues must be assessed. This will usually involve a planning meeting, around the 32nd week of the pregnancy (but not a formal care conference unless there are specific reasons). Here, the relevant professionals, including maternity and neonatal staff, can meet the parent or parents to identify problems, set goals and plan support networks. A decision on whether a formal care conference is required can also be made at this meeting. The case conference will then decide if a protection plan is needed.

The parents should be informed about all meetings and invited to attend.

4. Effects of drugs on the foetus and baby[9]

Studies examining the effects of illicit drugs in pregnancy are fraught with methodological difficulties. Small sample size, lack of obstetric information, and multiple confounding variables have produced inconsistent and sometimes contradictory findings. For the purposes of these Guidelines it is important to note that some of the effects of drug misuse during pregnancy are broadly similar and are largely non-specific. Intra-uterine growth retardation and pre-term deliveries contribute to increased rates of low birth-weight and increased perinatal mortality rate. These outcomes are multifactorial and are also affected by factors associated with socio-economic deprivation, including smoking.

Higher rates of early pregnancy loss and third-trimester placental abruptions appear to be major complications of maternal cocaine use. Increased rates of stillbirth, neonatal death[10] and sudden infant death syndrome[11] are found. Heroin appears to have a direct effect on foetal growth, with a higher rate of small-for-date noted babies, even when allowing for other confounding factors.

---

[9] Kaltenbach K., Finnegan L., 'Children of maternal substance misusers.' *Current Opinion in Psychiatry* 1997, **10**: 220–224.
[10] Chasnoff I.J., Burns W.J., Schnoll S.H., Burns K.A., 'Cocaine use in pregnancy.' *New England Journal of Medicine* 1985; **313**: 66–69.
[11] Kandall S.R., Gaines J., 'Maternal substance use and subsequent sudden infant death syndrome (SIDS) in offspring.' *Neurotoxicology and Teratology* 1991; **13**: 235–240.

5. Maternal health problems

There are a number of health problems in pregnancy which need to be discussed with the woman and reviewed throughout the pregnancy. These include general nutrition, risks of anaemia, dental hygiene and complications from chronic infection related to injection practice. These all contribute to the increased rate of obstetric complications and premature delivery found in drug-misusing women.

6. Management of labour

This is similar to any other woman, but pain relief needs special attention. Additional opiates may not be very effective if the receptors are already saturated. Therefore, there should be a low threshold for considering the use of an epidural. In addition, there may be increased placental insufficiency in pregnancies of drug-misusing women, leading to an increased risk of intrapartum hypoxia, foetal distress and meconium staining.

7. Neonatal withdrawal

Many babies will not need paediatric interventions, but it is important to have access to skilled neonatal paediatric care.

Signs of withdrawal from opiates are vague and multiple and tend to occur 24–72 hours after delivery. They include a spectrum of symptoms such as a high pitched cry, rapid breathing, hungry but ineffective sucking, and excessive wakefulness. At the other end of the spectrum symptoms include hypertonicity and convulsions but these are not common. Neonatal withdrawal can be delayed for up to 7–10 days if the woman is taking methadone in conjunction with benzodiazepines. Benzodiazepine use causes more prolonged symptoms, including respiratory problems and depression.

The drug treatment of neonatal withdrawal is outside the remit of these Guidelines.

8. Postnatal management

Breastfeeding should be encouraged, even if the mother continues to use drugs. The exceptions are: if she is HIV positive, because of the risk of HIV transfer when breastfeeding[12]; hepatitis C positive, because of the uncertainty around hepatitis C transmission; or where the mother uses a very high dose of benzodiazepines. Methadone treatment is not a contraindication to breastfeeding.

---

[12] Royal College of Obstetricians and Gynaecologists. *HIV infection in maternity care and gynaecology Revised report of the RCOG Sub-Committee on problems associated with AIDS in relation to obstetrics and gynaecology*. London: Royal College of Obstetricians, 1990.

9. Postnatal planning meeting

Soon after delivery, a meeting should be held to decide on the appropriate support for the mother from, for example, the social worker and the general practitioner, and whether extra supervision is necessary.

Health professionals should note that the care of the pregnant drug misuser and the safe delivery of the baby is just the start of care. Continuing support, which may need to include parenting advice and skills training, is essential after discharge if the ideal outcome of maintaining mother and child together is to be achieved.

For further information see: *Drug Using Parents: Policy guidelines for interagency working*, Local Government Drugs Forum and Standing Conference on Drug Abuse (1997). To order a copy call 0171 834 2222 quoting Local Association of Government reference SS084.

10. Prescribing drugs for pregnant drug misusers

Substitute prescribing can occur at any time in pregnancy. Conflicting advice to avoid the first trimester of pregnancy was based on pragmatic grounds, for example that a miscarriage at this stage, which occurs in all pregnancies at the rate of about one in five, would inadvertently be blamed on the prescribed medication.

a) Opiates[13]

Opiate treatment will depend on the general principles outlined in these Guidelines, with the additional point that it is better to keep a women in contact with services on low dose maintenance. The overall evidence indicates that low dose maintenance is the best option for ensuring continuity of management of pregnancy and aftercare. However, higher doses may be required if non-prescribed opiate use persists or recurs. Many mothers request detoxification. This option should be explored and their treatment goals and choice should be fully respected. Different drugs and regimes are available; however, methadone has been used safely for many years.[14, 15]

Generally, the principle of incremental reductions in methadone mixture to a level that minimises withdrawal in the mother and foetus should be pursued. A reasonable outpatient reduction regime would be to reduce methadone by 2.5–5mg weekly, fortnightly or monthly according to the woman's response. In the third trimester, many women will need an increase in methadone doses because of various physiological changes and weight gain. Dividing the daily dose can sometimes overcome the need for an increase in the dose in the later stages of pregnancy.

---

[13] Kaltenbach K., Berghella V., Finnegan L., 'Opioid dependence during pregnancy. Effects and management.' *Obstet Gynecol Clin North Am* 1998; **25**: 139–51.
[14] Schottenfeld R.S., 'Clinical trials of pharmacologic treatments in pregnant women – methadologic considerations.' *NIDA Research Monograph* 1995; **149**: 201–223.
[15] Finnegan L.P., Hagan T., Kaltenbach K.A., 'Scientific foundation of clinical practice: Opiate use in pregnant women.' *Bulletin of the New York Academy of Medicine* 1991; **67**: 223–239.

There is no clear dose relation between the intensity of neonatal withdrawal and maternal methadone dose at delivery[16], though studies have suggested that neonatal withdrawal reactions diminish with methadone dosages (of under 15mg), given at the time of delivery.

If detoxification is unsuccessful and the patient's drug use becomes uncontrolled, reduction could be stopped or the methadone dosage increased until stability is regained, so that detoxification and maintenance can be interchanged.

b) Cocaine

For those women using cocaine during their pregnancy, it is advised that they stop altogether, as there is no safe drug for substitute prescribing.[17]

11. Further reading

Drug Use in Pregnancy: Mother and Child, Chasnoff I.R. (ed.), MTP Press Limited, Falcon House. Lancaster, England, 1986.

Finnegan L.P., Kandall S.R., *Maternal and Neonatal Effects of Alcohol and Drugs, Substance Abuse: A Comprehensive Textbook*, J.H. Lowinson, P. Ruiz, R.B. Millman (eds), Baltimore, Maryland, Williams and Wilkins, 1992.

---

[16] Finnegan L.P., 'Neonatal abstinence', in Nelson N.M., (ed), *Current Therapy in Neonatal-Perinatal Medicine* 1990; Vol 2. Toronto: BC Dekker.

[17] Kaltenbach K., Finnegan L., 'Prevention and treatment issues for pregnant cocaine-dependent women and their infants.' *Ann NY Acad Sci* 1998; **846**: 329–334.

ANNEX 6
YOUNG PEOPLE AND DRUGS

Young people are defined for these Guidelines as those under 18 years.

1. Consent to treatment and the under 18s: the legal position

Young people aged 16–17 years

In England and Wales, minors aged 16 and 17 years can legally consent to any surgical, medical or dental treatment: the consent of a parent or guardian is not legally necessary.[1]

'Gillick Competent' children under 16 in England and Wales

Generally children under 16 years of age cannot legally give consent to treatment, and therefore consent needs to be obtained from a person with parental responsibility, usually a parent. However, a child under 16, with sufficient understanding and intelligence to fully comprehend what treatment is proposed, may also give legal consent to his or her treatment. Such a child is termed 'Gillick competent'.[2] The treating medical practitioner would have to decide whether or not a minor had sufficient intelligence and understanding to be Gillick competent.

Obtaining consent for procedures involving children and young people in Scotland

By virtue of the Age of Legal Capacity (Scotland) Act 1991, a person under the age of 16 years has legal capacity to consent on his/her own behalf to any surgical, medical or dental treatment, where, in the opinion of a qualified medical practitioner attending him/her, he/she is capable of understanding the nature and possible consequences of the procedure or treatment. In the majority of cases, children will be accompanied by their parents during consultation. Where, exceptionally, a child is seen alone, efforts should be made to persuade the child that his or her parents should be informed except in circumstances where it is clearly not in the child's best interests to do so. However, if a child capable of understanding the nature and consequences of the treatment refuses to allow their parent(s) or guardian(s) to be informed, the doctor should respect the rules of professional confidentiality. Parental consent should be obtained where a child under the age of 16 years does not have sufficient understanding, except in an emergency where there is no time to obtain it.

---

[1] Section 8 of the Family Law Reform Act 1969 makes this provision.
[2] *Gillick v West Norfolk and Wisbech Health Authority* 1985

Annex 6 Young People and Drugs

In the complex area of treating young drug misusers, these Guidelines recommend that, wherever possible, support for any proposed treatment is sought from an individual with parental responsibility. The likelihood of treatment being effective, will be greater if the treatment is undertaken with the acknowledgement and support of the young person's parents or guardian.

2. Principles of good practice

In addition to the general principles laid out in these guidelines, the following additional points should be taken into account when dealing with a young person who misuses drugs.

i)   All interventions should be undertaken in accordance with the guiding principle of the Children Act 1989, that the welfare of the child is paramount.

ii)   The practitioner should adhere to local policies and procedures that are agreed with the relevant local Area Child Protection Committee and Drug Action Team.

iii) The practitioner should involve other children's and young people's services and substance misuse services.

iv)   Family involvement should be seen as good practice.

v)   Interventions should follow a comprehensive assessment of need, developmental maturity, family factors and the risk of substance-related harm.

vi)   The provision of advice and treatment services separate to those from adults – that are both appropriate to and sensitive to the specific needs of children and young people in an environment appropriate to their age.

vii) If practitioners have concerns about issues of confidentiality, legal advice should be sought.

3. The role of services

In any locality there are a number of services which can provide assistance for young people using drugs, such as primary care, specialist alcohol and drug misuse treatment, child and adolescent health and mental health, and voluntary agencies.

Roles and responsibilities will differ according to the level of specialisation of the professionals involved. Primary care may provide information, advice, support, basic counselling and relapse prevention. Secondary care will provide more complex treatment interventions. In some situations an energetic outreach approach may be necessary, involving the resources of a multidisciplinary team. Any treatment plan should be fully explained and agreed with the child or young person and their parents where possible. It should have clear and measurable goals and be reviewed at regular intervals with the child or young person, their parents and other professionals involved. If other professionals are also involved with the child or young person, the doctor may need to take into account other care plans (educational and social services) the child or young person may have, and work with other professionals in a multidisciplinary shared care approach which dovetails health and social care planning.

4. Prescribing medication

Recommendations:

> **i)** As a person under the age of 16 is unlikely to have the capacity to understand the implications of being prescribed controlled drugs, doctors should avoid doing so unless they have first sought explicit consent from a person with parental responsibility for the young person.
>
> **ii)** Even with consent, the generalist or specialised generalist should only prescribe controlled drugs after a full assessment and supervision by a specialist.
>
> **iii)** Generalists, including child psychiatrists, should not prescribe substitute drugs without either specific training or formal liaison with a drug misuse treatment specialist.

In addition to the general principles and practice outlined elsewhere in the Guidelines, the following specific areas should be considered.

Careful assessment of indications to prescribe should take account of:

- Adverse effects directly relating to drug and alcohol misuse in young people largely result from intoxication.

- Drug misuse, even with some significant dependence, is not in itself an indication to prescribe substitute medication.

- Regular but not daily, non-dependent injecting of opiates is not necessarily an indication for prescribing substitute medication.

Opiate substitute prescribing should take account of the following points:

- It should follow the basic guidelines in Chapter 4.

- Longer-term or 'maintenance' prescribing is not recommended.

- The pharmacist should be informed in writing if a parent or guardian is to supervise the consumption of the drug. This arrangement should be agreed prior to the commencement of the prescription by all parties.

■ If possible, where family supervision is not available, daily supervised consumption should be arranged with the community pharmacist, with clear dispensing instructions.

5. Data collection and monitoring

Providers of services to young people must be prepared to establish much more comprehensive data collection and monitoring systems than would be the case with adults. These include:

■ recording all relevant issues on the service's user file at the time of initial assessment, including reasons for course of treatment chosen;

■ keeping written records of all contact with the young person and other agencies;

■ having policies and procedures for the sharing of information, and breaches in confidentiality, agreed with local agencies through the Area Child Protection Committee.

ANNEX 7
HIV AND HEPATITIS B AND C

1. HIV

a) Prevalence

Prevalence amongst intravenous drug misusers is about one in eighty for men and one in one hundred for women in London and the South East. Lower figures are found elsewhere in the United Kingdom. There is little evidence of current substantial HIV transmission through injecting drug use, though about 18 per cent of current intravenous drug misusers report recent sharing of equipment, and these rates are higher among young injectors and women.[1]

Figures in the UK are much lower than in other Western European countries of comparable size.[2]

b) Testing

HIV testing may be requested by drug misusers who perceive themselves to be at risk of having contacted the virus.

Issues to discuss before testing for any blood-borne virus should include:

- the likelihood of a positive test result;
- the potential social and financial implications of a positive result;
- the patient's understanding of what a positive test means medically;
- what supports are available to him or her;
- what forms of treatment might be available;
- results should ideally be given by the person who organised the test, as a planned consultation on a definite day;
- patients with positive results will need clear advice about onward medical treatment and referral.

Sometimes, an HIV test is requested immediately after an episode of high risk behaviour, such as needle sharing, and the patient needs to be advised that testing will not provide a reliable result until sufficient time has elapsed for the development of antibodies. A wait of three months between the last episode of risk-taking and the performing of the test is advisable, providing an accurate result in 99 per cent of all cases.

---

[1] Department of Health. *Unlinked anonymous HIV prevalence monitoring programme: England and Wales: data to the end of 1996: summary report from the Unlinked Anonymous Surveys Steering Group.* London: Department of Health, 1997.
[2] European Centre for the Epidemiological Monitoring of AIDS 1997. *HIV/AIDS Surveillance in Europe, Quarterly report no 55.*

If the patient tested for HIV:

- is found to be negative, reassure and advise about minimising future risk-taking; or

- is found to be positive, offer appropriate support, advice about how to avoid transmission to others, and offer referral for treatment. After learning of the diagnosis the drug misuser may become more chaotic and so will require considerable additional support.

The co-existence of HIV infection with drug misuse will, in many instances, have no effect on the management of the drug misuse by the patient. It is important to remember that an HIV-infected drug misuser who is asymptomatic may or may not be motivated to reduce their intake of, or come off, drugs. Do not make any assumptions.

For more details regarding drug use and HIV-infection refer to *Drug Use and HIV infection. The care of drug users and the treatment system*. WHO. Regional Office for Europe, Scherfigsvej 8. DK-2100 Copenhagen, Denmark.

2. Hepatitis B

Hepatitis B is transmitted parenterally and sexually. Transmission most commonly occurs following vaginal or anal intercourse or as the result of blood to blood contact, including sharing blood-contaminated needles and other injecting equipment by intravenous drug misusers, or by perinatal transmission from mother to child. The incubation period can vary between six weeks to six months, with the average period around three months. The severity of the illness varies from unapparent infections, which can only be detected by serological testing, to rare fulminating cases of acute hepatic necrosis. In adults, perhaps only about 30 per cent of acute infections result in jaundice and many cases may not be diagnosed.

About 5 per cent of immunocompetent adults infected with hepatitis B become chronic carriers of the virus, with hepatitis B surface antigen persisting for longer than six months. Among carriers of the virus, those in whom hepatitis B e-antigen is also detected are most infectious. Around 15–25 per cent of hepatitis B carriers may develop progressive liver disease, with an active hepatitis leading in some patients to cirrhosis. Chronic hepatitis B carriers with liver disease are at increased risk of developing hepatocellular carcinoma.

Hepatitis B surface antigen (HBsAg) is found in individuals with current infection, either acute or chronic; antibodies to hepatitis B core antigens (anti-HBc) are found in individuals with current or resolved infection; antibodies to hepatitis B surface antigen (anti-HBs) are found in those with previous resolved infections and following successful immunisation with hepatitis B vaccine. Recent cases of acute hepatitis B can be identified by testing for the IgM component of anti-core antibodies (anti-HBc IgM).

a) Immunisation

Hepatitis B vaccine is effective in preventing infection in individuals who produce specific antibodies to hepatitis B surface antigen (anti-HBs). Immunisation is recommended for injecting drug misusers not already infected or immune, and for the close household contacts, particularly the sexual partners, of any injecting drug misusers already infected. It is good practice to be proactive in offering immunisation to all these risk groups. Further information on dosage and immunisation schedules is given in the UK Health Department's memorandum *Immunisation against Infectious Disease 1996.*[3] Injecting drug misusers who are infected or already known to be immune will not require immunisation. It may be unwise to delay administration of the first dose of vaccine whilst awaiting test results; should a positive result then be obtained, it can be discussed with the user and immunisation discontinued. Where blood samples cannot be obtained, immunisation should proceed normally.

It is important to try to ensure that those being immunised receive three doses of vaccine.

b) Further management

Current and past injecting drug misusers who are infected with hepatitis B should be referred to a specialist with expertise in liver disease for further assessment, to determine what further management may be appropriate. They should also be given advice about their infectious state and on ways of reducing the risks of passing the infection to others, in particular the need to practice safer sex with partners not known to be immune.

3. Hepatitis C [4, 5]

The hepatitis C virus was first identified in 1989. Now that infections resulting from the transfusion of blood and blood products have largely been eliminated, the commonest route of transmission of hepatitis C in the UK is by sharing blood-contaminated needles or injecting equipment during intravenous drug misuse. Other parenteral routes capable of hepatitis C transmission via contaminated equipment include tattooing, body piercing and acupuncture. Sexual transmission occurs but the frequency is controversial, most studies indicate infection rates of less than 5 per cent in regular sexual partners, and a slightly increased seroprevalence in those with multiple sexual partners. Vertical (mother to baby) transmission appears to be of a similar order; there is thought to be increased risk of transmission if the mother has concomitant HIV infection.

Current evidence suggests that between 50 and 80 per cent of past and current injecting drug misusers may be infected with hepatitis C. Infection may often be acquired within the first six to twelve months of injecting, when sharing of injecting equipment may be more likely, and many injecting drug misusers may already have been infected by the time they access drug support services.

---

[3] Department of Health, Welsh Office, Scottish Home and Health Department, DHSS (Northern Ireland). *Immunisation against infectious disease.* London: HMSO, 1992; 110–119.
[4] Di Bisceglie A., 'Hepatitis C., *Lancet* 1998; **351**: 351–355.
[5] Booth J., Brown J., Thomas H., 'The management of chronic hepatitis C virus infection.' *GUT* 1995; **37**: 449–454.

Annex 7 HIV and Hepatitis B and C

The incubation period for hepatitis C virus is most commonly around six to nine weeks but can be longer; however, jaundice develops infrequently and most incident infections are unlikely to be diagnosed. It is currently thought that in the order of 20 per cent of new infections will resolve, whilst the virus will persist in around 80 per cent of cases. Although some of those with chronic hepatitis C infection experience vague, non-specific symptoms such as fatigue, aching joints etc, many will only develop symptoms later with the onset of complications of their liver disease. Virtually all patients with chronic hepatitis C will develop some inflammatory changes in the liver but these vary in severity. In some, the disease appears indolent and slowly progressive with a low grade of inflammation of the liver maintained for many years; others will have a much more active hepatitis, which in some may progress to cirrhosis. Around 20 per cent of patients with chronic infection are likely to develop cirrhosis, sometimes only after 20–30 years, and about 25 per cent of those with established cirrhosis may develop hepatocellular carcinoma (primary liver cancer) after a further period of time.

a) Testing

There are currently no screening tests to detect antigens of hepatitis C in the blood and evidence of infection is detected by testing for antibodies to the virus. These antibodies usually only become detectable late in the course of infection, but are likely to be present in most cases about three months after exposure. A negative result from a test performed within three months of the last exposure will not rule out infection, and testing should be repeated at an appropriate time. Tests for antibodies to hepatitis C virus (anti-HCV) do not distinguish between previous resolved, and established chronic, infection. Tests, performed in specialist centres, to detect the viral genome will determine which anti-HCV positive patients are viraemic.

Injecting drug users, both past and present, who have been at risk of exposure to hepatitis C and who seek testing should be offered well-informed advice and should be made aware of the implications of a positive test. Those who test negative should receive advice on ways of avoiding further exposure (there is no vaccine to protect against hepatitis C); those who test positive will need advice on ways of minimising the risks of transmitting infection to others.

b) Further management

It is essential to advise patients who are carrying the hepatitis C virus to avoid the use of alcohol.

All anti-HCV positive patients should be referred to a specialist with an interest in liver disease for confirmatory testing and further assessment. This will usually involve a period of observation and, in most cases, a liver biopsy, which helps to determine the level of inflammation and the stage of the disease. Patients with minimal disease will be kept under review, those considered to be at risk of progressive liver disease may be offered treatment with interferon. Although around half of patients respond initially to interferon, only 50 per cent of responders (i.e. 20–25 per cent of those treated) have a sustained response after cessation of treatment. In those showing an initial response to interferon, treatment is frequently continued for twelve months or more and requires significant commitment by the patient. Patients unable to comply with such a rigorous schedule (subcutaneous injections three times weekly, often self-administered) and the necessary attendance for monitoring of treatment, may be unsuitable for interferon therapy.

Other treatment approaches are under development, including the combination of interferon with other antiviral agents such as ribavirin.

c) For further information and facts refer to:

Strang J., Farrell M., *Hepatitis*, published by the Institute of the Study of Drug Dependence (ISDD), London, 1991; or
British Liver Trust. *Injecting Drug Use & Hepatitis C*, 1997. Information line 01473 276328.

ANNEX 8
ALCOHOL AND DRUG MISUSE

1. Introduction

Alcohol and drug misuse are commonly associated, especially amongst young drug misusers.[1]

It is beyond the scope of this section to outline guidelines for the full assessment and treatment of alcohol misuse and its related problems. There is, however, substantial evidence that brief interventions in a generic setting can have significant impact on drinking behaviour. General practitioners, nurses and other clinicians can play a public health role by regular screening and detection of excessive alcohol consumption and alcohol dependence, with follow-up advice to reduce consumption. Overall, clinicians tend to underestimate their capacity to impact on their patients' drinking behaviour.

For the purpose of these Guidelines, only details on alcohol detoxification are described. For more information on brief interventions and alcohol dependence please refer to:

Alcohol Concern's Brief Interventions Guidelines[2]
The Treatment of Drinking Problems. A Guide For the Helping Professionals[3]

2. Detoxification

For most patients' withdrawal, in-patient detoxification is not routinely required. Outpatient or home detoxification is often sufficient and has a good outcome in patients with a moderate alcohol withdrawal syndrome.[4]

For patients physically dependent on alcohol, planned detoxification may be appropriate, once it is established that the patient fulfils the following criteria:

■ No history of fits or delirium tremens
■ Not a suicide risk
■ Has social support
■ No significant polydrug misuse
■ Not dependent on benzodiazepines

[1] Parker H., Measham F., Aldridge J., *Drugs futures: changing patterns of drug use amongst English youth*. London: Institute for the Study of Drug Dependence, 1995.
[2] *Brief interventions guidelines*. Alcohol Concern, 1997.
[3] Edwards G., Marshall J., Cook C., *The Treatment of Drinking Problems. A Guide for the Helping Professionals*. 3rd Ed: Cambridge University Press, 1997.
[4] Collins M.N., Burns T., Van den Berk P., Tubman G., 'A structured programme for out-patient alcohol detoxification.' *British Journal of Psychiatry* 1990; **156**: 871–4.

If these criteria are not met, then inpatient detoxification with access to acute medical care is indicated.

After withdrawal, outpatient community treatment is appropriate.

A withdrawal plan should only be started if the patient is sober enough to agree the plan and understand the principles involved. The patient should agree not to take alcohol during the period of medication. Depending on the level of home support, daily visits to the home or outpatient clinic can be made to provide support and monitor progress. It is useful to give patients withdrawing at home an information leaflet.

a) Vitamin B

It is also useful to prescribe oral vitamin B complex or vitamin B_1 (thiamine) 50mg twice daily, for three weeks, to help in the recovery of thiamine levels. For those with the severe deficiency states, Wernickes's encephalopathy and Korsakoff's psychosis, intravenous or intramuscular administration of thiamine may be necessary. Intravenous injection should be given slowly over ten minutes. Facilities for treating anaphylaxis should be available when administered.

b) Benzodiazepines

> The use of chlormethiazole is not recommended as it induces dependence, and in overdose or in combination with alcohol may cause respiratory failure and coma.

Drug of choice – chlordiazepoxide (Librium) 10mg, though some experienced practitioners use diazepam.

The following chlordiazepoxide regime is recommended – though the dose level and length of treatment will depend on the severity of alcohol dependence and individual patient factors (e.g. weight, sex, liver function).

Day 1 & 2	20–30mg chlordiazepoxide QDS
Day 3 & 4	15mg chlordiazepoxide QDS
Day 5	10mg chlordiazepoxide QDS
Day 6	10mg chlordiazepoxide BD
Day 7	10mg chlordiazepoxide nocte

Dispensing should be daily, or involve the support of family members to prevent any risk of misuse or overdose. Confirm abstinence by checking for alcohol on the breath, or using a saliva test or breathalyser for three to five days.

It is best, if possible, to see the patient daily for the first five days and again after detoxification has finished. These do not need to be long consultations but they will allow the early detection of complications and encourage the patient to continue. Usually there will be a noticeable improvement in the patient as the detox progresses.

Where there is significant liver disease, diazepam and chlordiazepoxide metabolism is impaired, and it may be necessary to consider a benzodiazepine that is not metabolised in the liver, such as oxazepam.

c) Disulfiram 200mg (Antabuse)

Disulfiram is an alcohol sensitising agent that may be effective in helping some patients maintain abstinence. The success of this appears to be higher if the daily consumption of the drug is supervised. The disulfiram reaction includes flushing of the face, severe headaches, palpitations, nausea and vomiting. Large amounts of alcohol can produce arrhythmias, hypotension and collapse.

- Disulfiram can be used after a patient has undergone detoxification and wishes support in remaining alcohol free.
- It should only be initiated after a thorough assessment and requires careful monitoring.
- Alcohol should not be consumed for at least 24 hours before treatment.
- A normal dose is 800mg on the first day, reducing over 5 days to 200mg daily.

d) Acamprosate

More recently there is interest in the use of acamprosate as an anti-craving agent used in the maintenance of abstinence. There have been some initially promising results and it may become a useful adjunct to the current range of available services.[5]

3.   Non-drug interventions

Advice should be given on the location of Alcoholic Anonymous (AA) meetings, and patients should be encouraged to attend AA meetings as part of their initial treatment programme. Posters with information on NA and AA should be prominently displayed in patient waiting areas and leaflets on such programmes should be available. Knowledge of other local support groups and day programmes and active links with such programmes, can facilitate patient uptake.

---

[5] See the *British National Formulary* for more details.

ANNEX 9
THE CRIMINAL JUSTICE SYSTEM

1. Police custody

A large proportion of drug misusers come into conflict with the law and are taken into police custody. In that setting they may be seen by a police surgeon (forensic medical examiner) who has particular experience in assessing detainees for appropriate treatment. Forensic physicians should be clear as to their own guidelines.

In police stations where an arrest referral scheme operates, forensic medical examiners who suspect a detainee of drug misuse may wish to recommend that an arrested person is seen by an arrest referral worker for specialist assessment and advice.

2. The Probation Service

At least a third of individuals in contact with the Probation Service are drug misusers. In Scotland, responsibility for work with offenders in the community lies with the criminal justice arm of local authority social work departments.

The fact that an offender misuses drugs will be relevant to certain key probation functions:

- pre-sentence reporting and preparation of an outline supervision plan where a community sentence is proposed;

- providing information to help courts make bail decisions;

- supervision of community sentences, including those with treatment as a condition of probation;

- sentence planning and supervision of prisoners and ex-prisoners after release;

- referral to drug misuse treatment and advice agencies;

- referral to medical services within the prison and in the community.

Links with probation services can provide useful support and back-up and are available to most generalists for people who are currently on probation.

3. The new Drug Treatment and Testing Order (1998)

This order requires a consenting offender to undergo treatment for their drug problem, with regular testing to monitor compliance. The order will often be given in association with an existing community sentence, though in some instances it may stand alone. Since 1 October 1998, the Home Office has been piloting the order in parts of England (Croydon, Gloucestershire and Merseyside) to examine its effectiveness; a parallel pilot in Scotland is also taking place. The intention is to implement the strategy nationally after the pilots have run for 18 months.

4. The Prison Service

The prison population represents a good opportunity to access drug misusers for treatment and prevention work.

Since the Prison Service introduced its strategy for England and Wales, 'Drug Misuse in Prison', it has been making progress in introducing a range of treatment services for drug misusing offenders in prison, which now closely reflects those in the community. It published a revised Prison Service Strategy in May 1998[1]. The Scottish Prison Service published its policy on Drug Misuse in Prison in 1994, a revised version of which is expected in 1999.

The Prison Service also issues a set of standard health care procedures set out in *Health Care Standard 8*, regarding the appropriate use of prescribed substitute medication in the prison setting. *Health Care Standard 8* has been reviewed during 1998 with the intention of publishing it soon after the publication of these Clinical Guidelines.

It is recognised that prison is a unique operating environment with specific security requirements within which drug services have to be delivered safely and clinically responsibly. However, many of the principles of good practice laid out in Chapters 2 to 5 still apply in this context. Wherever possible, effective treatment established before imprisonment should be continued in the prison.

Doctors working within prisons should have the expertise and training to be able to provide the services of a specialised generalist (see Chapter 1).

Young offenders need special consideration in the light of awareness of increased suicidal risk in young prisoners with a history of alcohol and drug misuse. Women prisoners will require drug programmes that take their special needs into account.

It is recommended that drug misusers receive essential information on harm minimisation and have access to bleach. Ideally, they should receive immunisation against hepatitis B, if not already immune, and be warned of the risk of drug overdose on leaving prison, due to possible loss of tolerance. It is hoped that links with community services can promote continuity of care for reception into prison and for release into the community.

---

[1] *Tackling drugs in prison: The Prison Service drug strategy*. London: HM Prison Service 1998.

5. Recommended reading

Substance Misuse in Detainees in Police Custody. Guidelines for Clinical Management. Report of a Working Group. Department of Health, Scottish Office Home and Health Department, Welsh Office. London: HMSO.

ANNEX 10
ACCIDENT AND EMERGENCY

1. Introduction

For many drug misusers, accident and emergency (A&E) departments may be the first or only point of contact with health services, most often because of accidental overdoses and other crises.[1]

Aside from instances where they might be used in the management of severe pain, controlled drugs should only be prescribed in exceptional circumstances. These might include:

- opiate withdrawal in late pregnancy;

- concomitant physical/psychiatric illness where withdrawal might complicate the clinical picture;

- where admission is likely to be delayed for a considerable period of time.

Doctors should ensure that there are clear guidelines available for staff to respond to requests for medication (opiate and non-opiate) and injecting equipment.

As attendance at an A&E department may present a window of opportunity to put a drug misuser in touch with other services and consider his drug misuse, on discharge the following information should be given as a minimum:

- health promotion advice;

- contact points for further help.

Where available, the expertise of specialist liaison nurses or psychiatric/addiction services in the hospital should be used.

The patient's general practitioner should be informed of attendance.

---

[1] Gossop M., Marsden J., Edwards C., Wilson A., Segar G., Stewart D., Lehamann P., *The October Report: The National Outcome Research Study*. A Report Prepared For the Task Force 1995.

2. Overdose and suicides

> Hospital admission for the treatment of the medical complications of overdose should be considered in all cases.

Accidental overdose is not uncommon; 25 per cent of heroin users report having non-fatal accidental overdoses themselves[2] and 50 per cent report being present when another drug misuser has taken an overdose.[3] Overdose is more common within the first year of starting injecting use.

Diversion of prescribed methadone linctus is related to an increasing number of deaths amongst drug users.[4]

Accidental overdose is usually due to:

- varying purity of illicit supplies;
- reduction in tolerance after period of abstinence (e.g. release from prison, discharge from rehabilitation or hospital);
- mixing drugs (particularly injecting benzodiazepine, cocaine) and/or alcohol;
- leakage from poorly wrapped drugs that have been ingested (body stuffers and packers).

> Hospital admission for the treatment of medical complications of overdose should be considered in all cases but intoxication is not in itself sufficient grounds for compulsory admission under the Mental Health Act (1983).

a) Treatment

Emergency treatment should begin immediately professional help is available whether prior to or on admission to the accident and emergency department. All general measures (e.g. airway, breathing, circulatory support) should be instigated as necessary, alongside specific measures to treat the overdose.

Opiate overdose

If not in hospital, admit the patient.

> In most circumstances it should not be necessary to prescribe opiates or other controlled drugs for the management of addiction to a drug misuser in the A&E department.

---

[2] Gossop M., Griffiths P., Powis B., Williamson S., Strang J,. 'Frequency of non-fatal overdose: survey of heroin users recruited in non-clinical settings.' *British Medical Journal* 1996; **313**: 402.

[3] Darke S., Ross J., Hall W., 'Overdose among heroin users in Sydney, Australia: II. Responses to overdose.' *Addiction* 1996; **91**: 413–7.

[4] Cairns A., Roberts I.S., Benbow E.W., 'Characteristics of fatal methadone overdose in Manchester, 1985–94.' *British Medical Journal* 1996; **313**: 264–265.

Naloxone hydrochloride (Naloxone) is the antidote for opiate overdose. It is available as 1ml ampoules of 400 micrograms and as Min-I-Jet.

A dose at 0.8–2mg by intravenous injection should be administered, repeated at intervals of 2–3 minutes to a maximum of 10mg. If respiratory function does not improve, other diagnostic options such as other drug intoxication, or other organic causes of loss of consciousness including hypoglycaemia, should be considered.

The subcutaneous or intramuscular injection route should be used if an intravenous route is not accessible. The same regime should be employed as for intravenous use, but the clinician should expect a slower response.

Naloxone is short-acting, and repeated injections or intravenous infusion may be needed if a longer-acting opiate such as methadone has been taken. Naloxone can be given as a continuous intravenous infusion of 2mg diluted in a 500ml intravenous solution titrated at a rate determined by the clinical response.

The effects of methadone overdose can persist for up to 72 hours. Even in circumstances where patients have been resuscitated, depending on the magnitude of the overdose, they should be observed as an inpatient for a period of up to 72 hours. For high dose intoxication, naloxone infusion should be considered.

To enable rapid administration of naloxone prior to hospital admission, the following measures should be considered locally:

- GPs should carry naloxone in their emergency bag.

- Ambulance crew and paramedics should carry naloxone and should have clear protocols on the management of opiate overdose.

b) Management of other drugs

No antidote exists for the treatment of overdose from other drugs such as amphetamines, cocaine, cannabis, LSD and ecstasy. Treatment should therefore be aimed at the presenting symptoms and may include:

- management of the unconscious patient;

- management of hypothermia;

- management of acute psychosis.

ANNEX 11
MENTAL HEALTH

1. Drug misuse and co-morbid mental illness

There are increased rates of psychiatric disorders among those involved in heavy drinking and drug taking. Approximately one third of heavy drinkers have associated mental health problems and one-half of dependent drug takers have mental health problems of varying severity. Such mental health problems result in increased rates of service utilisation, poorer levels of social functioning and overall appear to be associated with poorer outcome. In the National Treatment Outcome Research Study, 29 per cent of the new admissions reported having suicidal thoughts in the previous three months and 10 per cent reported having a psychiatric hospital admission.[1]

There is increasing recognition that people in contact with general mental health services have increased rates of alcohol and drug problems, with approximately one-third reporting such problems.[2] These problems can also result in poorer outcome and greater levels of psychiatric hospitalisation.

These complex problems are heavily represented in populations such as the homeless and the prison population, where there are very high rates of alcohol and drug problems and also high rates of associated psychiatric disorder.[3]

2. General considerations

Medical professionals should regularly screen for, and be able to provide brief interventions for, anxiety and mood disorders in drug misusing patients. More severe cases of co-morbidity will usually require referral to a general psychiatrist, or a mental health specialist with special interest in drug misuse.

Patients with co-morbid mental illness are a particular challenge to emerging models of shared care, and at present there is considerable interest in the psychiatric and drug and alcohol misuse fields in drawing up guidelines for the joint management of these patients. There is a need for better models of liaison between Community Mental Health Teams, Community Substance Misuse Teams and Primary Care services, where an integrated multidisciplinary approach may improve and streamline overall service provision. Shared care between general psychiatrists, the general practitioner and a psychiatrist specialising in drug misuse is essential when planning an appropriate package of treatment. Many of these patients will have complex needs, requiring social services, the criminal justice system and housing agencies to provide input alongside medical services.

---

[1] Gossop M., Marsden J., Stewart D., *The National Treatment Outcome Research Study: changes in substance use, health and criminal behaviour one year after intake.* London: Department of Health, 1998.

[2] Menezes P.R., Johnson S., Thornicroft G., *et al.*, 'Drug and alcohol problems among individuals with severe mental illness in South London.' *British Journal of Psychiatry* 1996; **168**: 612–619.

[3] Farrell M., Howes S., Taylor C., *et al.*, 'Substance misuse and psychiatric comorbidity: an overview of the OPCS National Psychiatric Morbidity Survey.' *Addictive Behaviours* 1998; **23**: 909–918.

Although drug and alcohol dependence *per se* do not constitute grounds for compulsory admission to hospital, a patient may become so severely psychologically disturbed or suicidal as a result of taking drugs that treatment is essential to protect themselves or others. In these situations, compulsory treatment is justified and is permitted under the 1983 Mental Health Act in England and the Mental Health (Scotland) Act 1984.

3. Admission to a general psychiatric unit

The general principles of assessment and treatment are outlined in Chapters 2 to 4. In addition, clear operational policies to reduce the risk of illicit drug use on the ward and to help avoid disruptive behaviour and management problems must be in place. There should be a clear policy on follow-up, after both planned and unplanned discharge, and the conditions under which discharged patients can be re-admitted.

4. The homeless and prison population

The high rates of psychiatric morbidity and alcohol and drug dependence in the homeless require integrated management between the Community Mental Health Team, Substance Misuse Team and the Primary Care Team. Accommodation, albeit temporary, is often required before a patient can gain access to treatment facilities, so often, help to access hostel accommodation will be needed. Similarly, high rates for psychiatric morbidity and alcohol and drug dependence exist in the prison population.[4]

5. Continuing care

The general psychiatrist may need to act as the co-ordinator of care to ensure effective inter-disciplinary working. Many severely dependent drug misusers benefit from residential rehabilitation. However, many facilities will not accept people with a history of significant psychiatric disorders. The psychiatrist should develop a knowledge of what is available locally and establish good relationships with the relevant agencies.

6. Risk assessment

Risk assessment has become a significant responsibility for most of the helping professions. In the context of risk assessment, a full and comprehensive history of alcohol and drug use and its relationship to episodes of violence is essential.[5,6] The role of alcohol and drugs in precipitating episodes of severe mental illness and also in aggravating risks of serious offending, needs to be fully enquired about and carefully documented to ensure adequate communication within the multidisciplinary team.

7. Care Pathway Approach (CPA)

In England, patients with significant mental illness should be treated under CPA with a named key worker. Those with complex needs should be managed under a higher CPA regime, with regular meetings of involved professionals, patients and carers.

[4] Singleton N., Meltzer H., Gatward R., Coid J., and Deasy D., *Psychiatric morbidity among prisoners in England and Wales*. London: The Stationery Office. 1998.

[5] Wallace C., Mullen P., Burgess P., Palmer S., Ruschena D. and Browne C., 'Serious criminal offending and mental disorder.' *British Journal of Psychiatry* 1998; **172**: 477–484.

[6] Johns A., 'Substance misuse: a primary risk and a major problem of co-morbidity.' *International Review of Psychiatry* 1997; **9**: 233–241.

Annex 11 Mental Health

ANNEX 12
HARM MINIMISATION FOR INJECTING DRUG MISUSERS

The first principle of minimising harm should be to stop injecting practice.

The ramifications of sharing any injecting equipment (spoons, water, filters, needles, syringes etc.) must be addressed with every misuser.

As drug misusers will inevitably resort to cleaning of equipment, it is good practice to advise them of the best method they might follow, even allowing for its potential risks.

1. The importance of sterile injecting equipment

Injecting drug misuse carries a significant risk of infection, particularly when equipment is shared or cursorily cleaned. Dirty and unhygienic injecting habits can result in local or systematic infections, and poor injecting technique can cause venous or arterial thrombosis.

Nearly all localities have organised provision for accessing sterile injecting equipment, either through pharmacy-based needle exchange, or other forms of needle exchange. Information on these services should be available to those who are injecting drugs and at risk of injecting drugs. Injectors should be informed of the dangers of using used injecting equipment, and encouraged to be scrupulous in their hygiene technique if injecting drugs. They should be advised to use sterile or at least their own equipment on each occasion, if they are to reduce their risk of acquiring hepatitis C, B or HIV.

The harm associated with injection can be reduced by advising about poor injecting technique, providing clean needles and syringes, and by giving correct advice on cleaning injecting equipment.[1] Most significantly, the sharing of needles, syringes and injection equipment (spoons, filters, water) needs to be clearly addressed with the patient. Many drug misusers only consider sharing to be the joint use of the needle or syringe and have not considered that water used for preparation and disposal, and other injecting paraphernalia such as filters, can also run significant contamination risks, and possibly play a significant role in the transmission not only of HIV, but also of the hepatitis B and C viruses.

---

[1] Stimson G., Aldritt L., Dolan K., Donaghue N., Lart R., *Injecting equipment exchanges schemes: final report*. London: Goldsmiths College, 1988.

2. Safer injecting use

■ Always inject with the blood flow.

■ Rotate injection sites.

■ Use sterile new injecting equipment, with the smallest-bore needle possible.

■ Avoid neck, groin, breast, feet and hand veins.

■ Mix powders with sterile water and filter solution before injecting.

■ Always dispose of equipment safely (either in a bin provided or by placing the needle inside the syringe and placing both inside a drinks can).

■ Avoid injecting into infected areas.

■ Do not inject into swollen limbs, even if the veins appear to be distended.

■ Poor veins indicate a poor technique. Try to see what is going wrong.

■ Do not inject on your own.

■ Learn basic principles of first aid and cardiopulmonary resuscitation in order that you may help friends at times of crisis.

3. Cleaning injecting equipment

It is best to always use sterile needles and syringes each time. Although cleaning equipment is a safer practice than not cleaning at all, there is no absolutely certain way of cleaning needles, syringes and drug paraphernalia that will guarantee no infection risk. Such practice is of course less secure when paraphernalia are still being shared, or not adequately cleaned.

The advice about cleaning injecting equipment has only been shown to reduce the risk of HIV and may offer *little or no protection* against the more enduring and prevalent hepatitis C.

The following table summarises how to clean needles and syringes with undiluted household bleach.

Cleaning injecting equipment

The following are needed to bleach clean injecting equipment:

- Needle and syringe

- Thin, undiluted household bleach

- Clean, cold water

- Two clean cups, or wide-topped bottles

Method

1. Pour bleach into one cup (or bottle) and water into another.

2. Draw bleach up with the dirty needle and syringe.

3. Expel bleach into sink.

4. Repeat steps 2 and 3.

5. Draw water up through needle and syringe.

6. Expel water into sink.

7. Repeat steps 5 and 6 at least two or three times.

Points to remember when cleaning equipment

- Boiling plastic syringes melts them.

- Thick bleach is impossible to draw up through a needle.

- Cold water is recommended as warm water may encourage blood to coagulate and hence will be harder to expel through the needle.

4. Other administration routes

It is important to advise non-injectors that snorting (nasal inhalation), smoking or swallowing drugs, though safer than injection, are not administration routes entirely without risk. Hot smoke, if not cooled first, can damage bronchial tissues, and inhaled heroin or cocaine can precipitate asthma. Inhaled cocaine is also associated with bronchitis, pneumothorax, pulmonary oedema, and obliterative bronchiolitis.[2]

Nasal inhalation, sniffing or snorting is normally associated with powdered cocaine and amphetamine, Prolonged use of cocaine in this way can cause atrophy of the nasal septum and breathing problems.

The simplicity of oral drug use increases the use of experimentation, either through mixing drugs or taking large quantities. The possibility of risk of overdose from cocktails of drugs, especially when taken with alcohol, cannot be overestimated.

Sensible advice to the non-injector to minimise the harm of drug misuse would include the following:

i)   Know what you are taking.

ii)   Using cocktails of drugs can be more dangerous than single drug use.

iii)   It is dangerous to mix drugs and alcohol.

iv)   Look after yourself (eat, sleep, exercise and rest sufficiently).

---

[2] Khalsa M-E., Tashkin D., Perrochet B., 'Smoked cocaine: patterns of use and pulmonary consequences.' *Journal of Psychoactive Drugs* 1992; **24**: 265–272.

ANNEX 13
HOW TO WRITE A PRESCRIPTION FOR A CONTROLLED DRUG

A prescription must be signed and dated by the prescriber and specify the prescriber's address. A prescription is valid for 13 weeks from the date stated.

The prescription must always state in the prescriber's own handwriting in ink or otherwise so as to be indelible:

i)   the patient's name and address;

ii)   in the case of a preparation, the form (even when it is implicit in the proprietary name or where only one form is available) and, where appropriate, the strength of the preparation (where more than one strength exists the strength required must be specified);

iii)   the total quantity of the preparation (the number of dose units) in **both** words and figures (this does not apply to temazepam);

iv)   the dose;

v)   be signed and dated by the prescriber.

If the starting date is other than the date of writing the prescription then this should be clearly stated on the prescription. Otherwise prescriptions can legally only be dispensed starting from the date written.

A prescription does not have to be in the prescriber's own handwriting in ink when:

i)   it is a prescription for temazepam;

ii)   the prescriber has been specifically exempted from this requirement;

iii)   the prescription contains no controlled drug other than phenobarbitone or phenobarbitone sodium or a preparation containing either of these;

iv)   the exemption does **not** apply to the date. A computer-generated date need not be deleted, but the date must also be added by the prescriber.

A prescription may order a controlled drug to be dispensed by instalments; the amount of the instalments and the intervals to be observed must be specified. Prescriptions ordering 'repeats' on the same form are **not** permitted.

A special form, FP10(HP)(ad), in Scotland HBP(A), is available to doctors in NHS drug treatment centres for prescribing cocaine, dextromoramide, diamorphine, dipipanone, methadone, morphine or pethidine by instalments for addicts. In Scotland, general practitioners can prescribe by instalments from GP10. In England and Wales, forms FP10 and FP10(HP) are not suitable for this purpose but form FP10(MDA) is available and is generally used for no more than 14 instalments.

In all cases, a licence is necessary to prescribe cocaine, diamorphine or dipipanone for addicts, except for treatment of organic disease or injury.

ANNEX 14
DRUG INTERACTIONS

Methadone drug interactions

Drug	Status of interaction	Effect	Mechanism
Alcohol	Clinically important.	Increased sedation, increased respiratory depression. Combination may also have increased hepatotoxic potential.	Additive central nervous system depression.
Barbiturates	Clinically important.	Reduced methadone levels. Increased sedation. Additive CNS depression.	Barbiturates stimulate hepatic enzymes involved in methadone metabolism.
Benzodiazepines	Clinically important.	Enhanced sedative effect.	Additive CNS depression.
Buprenorphine	Clinically important.	Antagonist effect or enhanced sedative and respiratory depression.	Buprenorphine is a partial agonist of opiate receptors.
Carbamazepine	Clinically important.	Reduced methadone levels.	Carbamazepine stimulates hepatic enzymes involved in methadone metabolism.
Chloral hydrate	Clinically important.	Enhanced sedative effect.	Additive CNS depression.
Chlormethiazole	Clinically important.	Enhanced sedative effect.	Additive CNS depression.

Drug	Status of interaction	Effect	Mechanism
Cimetidine	Two cases have been shown in patients taking methadone as analgesia.	Possible increase in methadone plasma levels.	Cimetidine inhibits hepatic enzymes involved in methadone metabolism.
Cisapride Domperidone Metoclopramide	Theoretical.	Theoretically might increase the speed of onset of methadone absorption, but not the extent.	Possibly by reversing the delayed gastric emptying associated with opioids.
Cyclizine and other sedating anti-histamines.	Clinically important.	Anecdotal reports of injection of cyclizine with opiates causing hallucinations. Reports of injection of high doses of dephenhydramine with opiates to achieve 'buzz'.	Additive psychoactive effects. Anti-muscarinic effects at high doses.
Desipramine*	Clinically important.	Raised desipramine levels by up to a factor of two.	Unknown interaction not seen with other tricyclic antidepressants.
Other tricyclic antidepressants	Theoretical.	Enhanced sedative effect, which is dose dependent.	Additive CNS depression.
Disulfiram	Avoid in combination with methadone formulations containing alcohol (check with manufacturers).	Very unpleasant reaction to alcohol which can be alarming.	Disulfiram inhibits alcohol metabolism. allowing metabolites to build up.
Erythromycin	In theory should interact, but combination has not been studied.	Increase in methadone levels.	Decreased methadone metabolism.

Drug	Status of interaction	Effect	Mechanism
Fluconazole	In theory the same as ketoconazole.		
Fluoxetine	Clinically important.	Raised methadone levels, but not as significant as for fluvoxamine.	Decreased methadone metabolism.
Fluvoxamine	Clinically important.	Raised plasma methadone levels.	Decreased methadone metabolism.
Other SSRI	Theoretical.		
Grapefruit Juice	Should interact in theory and there have been several anecdotal reports.	Raised methadone levels.	Decreased methadone metabolism.
Indinavir	Clinically important.	Raised methadone levels.	Decreased methadone metabolism.
Ketoconazole	Clinically important.	Raised methadone levels.	Decreased methadone metabolism.
MAOI (including selegiline and moclobemide)	Severe with pethidine though unlikely with methadone and has never been described.	CNS excitation delirium, hyperpyrexia, convulsions, hypotension or respiratory depression.	Unclear. Avoid the combination if possible.
Naltrexone	Clinically important.	Blocks effect of methadone (long acting)	Opiate antagonist – competes for opiate receptors.
Naloxone	Clinically important.	Blocks effect of methadone (short acting), but may be needed if overdose suspected.	Opiate antagonist – competes for opiate receptors.

Drug	Status of interaction	Effect	Mechanism
Nevirapine	Clinically important.	Decreased methadone levels.	Increased methadone metabolism.
Nifedipine	Has been demonstrated *in vitro* only.	Increased nifedipine levels. No effect on methadone levels.	Methadone increases the metabolism of nifedipine.
Omeprazole	To date, demonstrated only in animals.	Increased methadone levels.	Possibly an effect upon methadone absorption from the gut.
Phenobarbitone	See barbiturates above.		
Phenytoin	Clinically important.	Reduced methadone levels.	Phenytoin stimulates hepatic enzymes involved in methadone.
Rifampicin	Very important: most patients are likely to affected.	Reduced methadone levels.	Rifampicin stimulates hepatic enzymes involved in methadone metabolism.
Rifabutin	Occasionally clinically important.	Decreased methadone levels.	Increased methadone metabolism.
Ritonavir	Clinically important.	Ritonavir may increase plasma methadone levels.	Inhibits methadone metabolism.
Other protease inhibitors	Theoretical.	May raise or lower methadone plasma levels.	Inhibits methadone metabolism.
Urine acidifiers e.g. ascorbic acid – vitamin C	Clinically important.	Reduced plasma methadone levels.	Raised urinary excretion of methadone.

Drug	Status of interaction	Effect	Mechanism
Urine alkalinisers e.g. sodium bicarbonate	Clinically important.	Increased plasma methadone levels.	Reduced urinary excretion of methadone.
Zidovudine	Clinically important.	Raised plasma levels of zidovudine. No effects on methadone levels.	Unknown.
Zopiclone	Clinically important.	Enhanced sedative effect.	Additive CNS depression.
Other opiates	Clinically important.	Enhanced sedative effect. Enhanced respiratory depression.	Additive CNS depression.
Other CNS depressant drugs (e.g. neuroleptics, hyoscine)	Clinically important.	Enhanced sedative effect, which is dose dependent.	Additive CNS depression.

* Desipramine is only available on a named patient basis.

Adapted from: Preston A., *The Methadone Briefing*, ISDD: London, 1996.

Additional material and advice from Simon Wills, head of Drug Information, St Mary's Hospital, Portsmouth, and the *British National Formulary*.

ANNEX 15
CONVERSION TABLE

Drug	Dose	Methadone equivalent
Street Heroin	Cannot accurately be estimated because street drugs vary in purity, though 1g of street heroin is roughly equivalent to 50–80mg oral methadone. Titrate dose against withdrawal symptoms.	
Pharmaceutical Heroin	10mg tablet or 30mg ampoule	20mg 60mg
Methadone	10mg ampoule Mixture (1mg/ml) 10ml Linctus (2mg/5ml) 10ml	10mg 10mg 4mg
Morphine	10mg ampoule	10mg
Dipipanone (Diconal)	10mg tablet	4mg
Dihydrocodeine (DF118)	30mg tablet	3mg
Dextromoramide (Palfium)	5mg tablet 10mg tablet	5–10mg 10–20mg
Pethidine	50mg tablet 50mg ampoule	5mg 5mg
Buprenorphine hydrochloride (Temgesic or Subutex)	200 microgram sublingual tablet 400 microgram sublingual tablet 300 microgram ampoule New formulations – 2mg and 8mg sublingual tablets	5mg 10mg 8mg Methadone equivalents are not currently available
Pentazocine (Fortral)	50mg capsule 25mg tablet	4mg 2mg

Drug	Dose	Methadone equivalent
Codeine linctus 100ml	300mg codeine phosphate	20mg
Codeine phosphate	15mg tablet 30mg tablet 60mg tablet	1mg 2mg 4mg
Gee's linctus 100ml	16mg anhydrous morphine	10mg
J. Collis Brown 100ml	10mg extract of opium	10mg

These conversions do not necessarily suffice for daily requirements because of the different half-lives of drugs.

ANNEX 16
DRUGS AND DRIVING

1. Driving licence requirements

The Driver and Vehicle Licensing Agency (DVLA) has recently made available a new edition of their 'At a glance Guide' which sets out the medical standards that are required for the holding of licences.[1] This document outlines the new regulation on persistent misuse of drugs.

Under the terms of the Road Traffic Act, holders of a driving licence are required to inform the Driver and Vehicle Licensing Authority (DVLA) of " . . . any disability likely to affect safe driving".

According to the DVLA, drug use, whether or not amounting to dependency, is regarded as a disability in this context. Additionally, the use of prescribed medication to treat drug/substance misuse constitutes a relevant disability.

This responsibility lies with the holder, not the prescribing doctor or drug service.

A patient with a Group 1 driving licence will be required to undergo a short independent medical examination which will include a urine screen for drugs. If there are only methadone metabolites in the urine, a licence will usually be issued for one year at a time, until three years have elapsed since the cessation of treatment. The issue of a licence is subject to the fact that the person is on a supervised methadone withdrawal course and is supported by a favourable consultant report.

If the patient informs the DVLA that they are receiving injectable, as opposed to oral, methadone on prescription, the licence is likely to be withdrawn. However, a letter from a consultant psychiatrist confirming that the patient experiences low levels of sedation, may exceptionally result in a decision to treat the prescription of injectable methadone in the same way as oral methadone.

On re-application, the patient will have to undergo a medical; this will include a urine screen for drugs. They will be called back for another medical every year until three years after methadone treatment has finished.

---

[1] Driver and Vehicle Licensing Agency., *At a glance guide to medical aspects of fitness to drive*. Swansea: DVLA, 1998. The guide has been sent to all GP surgeries. Further information can be obtained from:

The Senior Medical Adviser
DVLA
Driver Medical Unit
Longview Road
Morriston
Swansea
SA99 1TU

DVLA will not issue a Group 2 (HGV/PSV) to anyone receiving methadone treatment. A patient with a Group 2 (HGV/PSV) licence, who informs the DVLA that they are receiving methadone on prescription, will have that licence withdrawn for a minimum of three years.

If a urine screen carried out for a DVLA medical examination shows persistent misuse of cannabis, the DVLA will withdraw the licence for one year. If it shows positive for any other drug, they will withdraw the licence for a minimum of one year, but this may be up to three years in cases of persistent misuse. There will be another medical on re-application and every year for the first three years after the licence has been returned.

2. Driving under the influence of drugs

It is an offence to be in charge of a vehicle if "unfit to drive through drink or drugs".

A patient taking a prescribed drug like methadone would not automatically be considered by the courts to be unfit to drive.

Whether or not practitioners should take the step of breaching confidence and informing the DVLA without their patient's consent, if they are concerned about their patient's ability to drive or if the patient is driving passenger or heavy goods vehicles, is a complex but real ethical issue.

The General Medical Council's code states that doctors "should explain to patients that they have a legal duty to inform the DVLA. If the patient refuses to accept the diagnosis or the effect of the condition, you can suggest that the patient seeks a second opinion. You should advise patients not to drive until the second opinion has been obtained. If patients continue to drive . . . you should make every reasonable effort to persuade them to stop. This may involve telling their next of kin. If you do not manage to persuade patients to stop driving, or you are given or find evidence that a patient is continuing to drive contrary to advice, you should disclose relevant medical information immediately, in confidence, to the medical adviser at the DVLA. Before giving information to the DVLA you should inform the patient of your decision to do so. Once the DVLA has been informed, you should also write to the patient, to confirm that a disclosure has been made."

ANNEX 17
TRAVELLING ABROAD

1. Travelling with Methadone

a) Amounts less than 500mgs

Drug misusers in receipt of a prescription for methadone can travel abroad with their supply. A Home Office licence is not necessary for amounts of up to 500mgs.

However, the Home Office advise travellers to carry a 'To whom it may concern' letter from the prescriber, indicating that they are in possession of the drug for legitimate medical purposes.

b) Amounts over 500mgs

For amounts over 500mgs a Home Office licence is required. The prescriber must write to the Home Office stating:

- the name and address of the person
- the strength
- the form
- the quantity of the drug
- the daily rate prescribed
- the person's date of departure and return.

There is nothing laid down about the maximum amounts that individuals may travel with and the Home Office advises that each case is treated on its merits.

The licence is to take the drug out of the UK and to bring any surplus back in. **It does not mean that the holder of the licence has the right to take the drug into the country to be visited**. Therefore, it is important that the user checks with the embassy or consulate before departure, to establish that the country/countries to be visited will accept the Home Office licence.

Anyone applying for a licence should allow at least seven working days, if all the information needed is contained in the letter from the prescriber, for the processing of the application.

A licence is obtainable from:

Home Office Drugs Branch
Licensing Section
Room 239
Queen Anne's Gate
London
SW1H 9AT

> **The requirements laid out above are similar for all/most prescribed drugs contained in Schedules 2 and 3 of the Misuse of Drugs Regulations 1985.**

For further information, contact the Home Office at the above address, or telephone 0171 273 3806.

ANNEX 18
MONITORING PROGRESS AND OUTCOMES OF TREATMENT

Monitoring activity is the process of collecting information to allow an assessment of whether or not goals have been met, or assessment of progress towards these goals.

Monitoring can occur at any level of care, from the individual doctor, primary health care team within a practice, to the level of a primary care group (or equivalent), or at the level of a health authority or health board.

Monitoring progress and outcomes of treatment within case management

Some monitoring activity will occur routinely during a consultation as the GP or drugs worker records the patient's progress against treatment goals. Chapter 4, 'The Responsibilities and Principles of Prescribing for Drug Dependence' discusses goal setting and record keeping as part of prescribing for drug dependence.

Monitoring activity may include use of specific indicators such as the results of urine analysis. Methods of urinalysis are described in Chapter 3, 'Assessment'. Doctors may also wish to consider the use of specific instruments, which have been developed to assist in assessment of progress and outcomes of treatment, such as the Addiction Severity Index[1], the Opiate Treatment Index[2] or the instrument developed for use by the National Treatment Outcome Research Study.[3] The Maudsley Addiction Profile (MAP)[4] is a brief, interviewer-administered questionnaire to record recent problems experienced by adult drug (and alcohol) users; it is the only instrument of the above three that has been developed for and in Britain.

The MAP is designed to be easily administered at the stages of initial assessment and after a period of treatment. The questionnaire takes about 12 minutes to complete and is divided into four sections covering substance use, health risk behaviour, physical and psychological health and personal social functioning. The MAP is a research instrument that can be used free of charge for non-profit-making organisations.[5]

---

[1] McLellan A.T., Luborsky L., O Brien C.P., Woody G.E., 'An improved evaluation instrument for substance abuse patients.' *Journal of Nervous and Mental Diseases* 1980; **168**: 26–33.

[2] Darke S., Hall W., Wodak A., Heather N., and Ward J., Development and validation of a multidimensional instrument for assessing outcome of treatment among opiate users: the Opiate Treatment Index.' *British Journal of Addiction* 1992; **87**: 733–742.

[3] Gossop M., Marsden J., Stewart D., *National Treatment Outcome Research Study*. London: Department of Health, 1997.

[4] The Maudsley Addiction Profile

[5] Information on the MAP and its use can be obtained from Dr John Marsden at the Addiction Research Unit, Maudsley Hospital/Institute of Psychiatry, 4 Windsor Walk, London, SE5 8AF.

Annex 18 Monitoring Progress and Outcomes of Treatment

Monitoring outcomes of treatment at a local level

Chapter 2, 'Treatment' describes the role of monitoring groups in shared care arrangements. The monitoring group may, as part of its work, approve local development schemes, payment arrangements for practitioners, guidelines and protocols, and clarify performance indicators.

Performance indicators identified by the Task Force to Review Services for Drug Misusers

Annex H of the report *Task Force to Review Services for Drug Misusers* suggests a number of performance indicators which may be applied in primary care settings.[6] While the choice of measures and standards to be set is for local determination, the Task Force considered those highlighted in bold as the most appropriate for initial consideration.

- ■ Percentage of specialist service clientele registered with a GP.

- ■ Percentage of participating GPs with clear guidelines for 'shared care', including well-defined liaison arrangements.

- ■ **Percentage of GPs prepared to take or undertaking shared care responsibilities.**

- ■ **Percentage of specialist drug service clients cared for in general practice.**

- ■ Costs per GP-managed client.

Health authority monitoring of drug misuse treatment in primary care settings

Recent guidance from the Department of Health to health authorities[7], about the funding of drug misuse services from 1999/2000, describes primary care as the ideal setting to offer treatment both for basic health needs of drug users and problems associated with drug misuse. It describes indicative targets for health authorities to meet by the end of 1999/2000. These include an increase in the number of drug misusers receiving treatment in primary care settings and that the proportion of GPs who treat drug misusers in any health authority should be at least 20 per cent. Health authorities will be expected to monitor performance with respect to these targets, reporting progress through local Drug Action Teams and through returns to the Regional Drug Misuse Database.

The guidance also suggests that health authorities may wish to monitor performance of drug misuse treatment through use of the performance indicators listed in Annex H of the *Task Force to Review Services for Drug Misusers*. Monitoring arrangements in Scotland are being considered separately within the context of Scotland's enhanced strategy *Tackling Drugs in Scotland: Action in Partnership*.

---

[6] Department of Health. *Task Force to review services for drug misusers: report of an Independent Review of Drug Treatment Services in England*. London: Department of Health, 1996. (Chairman: The Reverend John Polkinghorne)
[7] Health Service Circular. Number HSC 1999/036. *Drug Misuse Special Allocation: 1999/2000. Funding and Guidance on the Modernisation Fund Element*.

ANNEX 19
REFERENCES AND CONTACT NUMBERS

1. Regional Drug Misuse Databases

a) England

Anglia and Oxford
Telephone 01865 226734; fax 01865 226652

North West
Merseyside and Cheshire: telephone 0151 794 5774; fax 0151 794 5488
North Western: telephone 0161 772 3782; fax 0161 772 3445

Northern and Yorkshire
Telephone 0113 295 1337; fax 0113 295 1310

South and West (including Wessex)
South Western: telephone 0117 9958 4384; fax 0117 958 6569

North Thames/South Thames
Telephone 0181 846 6563; fax 0181 846 6555

Trent
Telephone 0116 286 3267; fax 0116 275 2840

West Midlands
Telephone 0121 695 2347; fax 0121 695 2349

b) Scotland:

The Scottish Drug Misuse Database
Telephone 0131 551 8715; fax 0131 551 1392

c) Wales

Telephone 01222 667 766; fax 01222 665 940

d) Northern Ireland

In Northern Ireland, the Misuse of Drugs (Notification of and Supply to Addicts) (Northern Ireland) Regulations 1973 require doctors to send particulars of persons whom they consider to be addicted to certain controlled drugs to the Chief Medical Officer of the Department of Health and Social Services. The Northern Ireland contacts are:

Medical contact: Administrative contact:

Senior Medical Officer   Health Promotion Branch
C3.9 Castle Buildings   C4.22 Castle Buildings
Belfast BT4 3PP   Belfast BT4 3PP

Telephone 01232 520170   Telephone 01232 520532

2.   Other contact numbers:

ADFAM National
(National Charity for the Families and Friends of Drug Misusers)
Waterbridge House
32–36 Loman Street
London SE 1 0EE
Tel 0171 928 8900
Fax 0171 928 8923

Alcohol Concern
Waterbridge House
32–36 Loman Street
London SE1 0EE
Tel 0171 928 7377
Fax 0171 928 4644

Association of Nurses in Substance Abuse
120 Wilton Park Road
London SW1V 1JZ
Tel 0171 233 8322
Fax 0171 233 7779

Drugs in School Helpline
Release
388 Old Street
London EC1 V 9IT
Tel 0345 366666
Fax 0171 729 2599

Health Eduction Authority (HEA)
Trevelyan House
30 Great Peter Street
London SW1P 2HW
Tel 0171 383 3833 (Health promotion information service)
Fax 0171 387 0660

Drug Prevention Advisory Service
Home Office
Horseferry House
Dean Ryle Street
London SW1P 2AW
Tel 0171 217 8631

Institute for the Study of Drug Dependence (ISDD)
Waterbridge House
32–36 Loman Street
London SE1 0EE
Tel 0171 803 4720
Website: www.isdd.co.uk

Narcotics Anonymous (NA)
UK Service Office
PO Box 1980
London N19 3LS
Helpline 0171 730 0009
Publications 0171 272 9040

National Drugs Helpline
Tel 0800 776600
Provides 24-hour free and confidential advice, including information on local services.

Royal Pharmaceutical Society of Great Britain
1 Lambeth High Street
London
SE1 7JN
Tel 0171 735 9141
Fax 0171 735 7629

Substance Misuse Advisory Service (SMAS)
46–48 Grosvenor Gardens
London
SW1W 0EB
Tel 0171 881 9255
Fax 0171 881 9260

Standing Conference on Drug Abuse (SCODA)
Waterbridge House
32–36 Loman Street
London SE1 0EE
Tel 0171 928 9500
Fax 0171 928 3343

TACADE
(Advisory Council on Alcohol and Drug Education)
1 Hulme Place
The Crescent
Salford
Manchester M5 4QA
Tel 0161 745 8925
Fax 0161 745 8923

To find out the contact details for the nearest Drug Action Team, see the ISDD website (given above) or telephone/email the UK Anti-Drugs Coordination Unit on 0171 270 6057/ ukadcu@gtnet.gov.uk.